Loving Living Gluten Free

Recipes That Work

Kathy A Babbitt

AuthorHouse™
1663 Liberty Drive
Bloomington, IN 47403
www.authorhouse.com
Phone: 1 (800) 839-8640

Published by AuthorHouse 12/17/2016

ISBN: 978-1-5246-5382-8 (sc)
ISBN: 978-1-5246-5381-1 (e)

Library of Congress Control Number: 2016920221

Print information available on the last page.

This book is printed on acid-free paper.

authorHOUSE®

Contents

Dedication

This book is the culmination of a lifetime of work, the last 11 years working with recipes and formulas trying to normalize life without gluten. I cannot possibly name all the taste testers, critics (thank God for them!) and my champions.

I would like however to signal out a few. **God,** for which all things are possible and all gifts are given. My husband **Scott Babbitt,** for this would have not been possible without him and his support. He provides for us a wonderful life that enables me to live out my dream. **Scott & Donna Babbitt** for proofing this book, and all their encouragement! **Vicky Scherberger,** your leadership training from Executive Leadership Skills International gave me confidence to do all I have been able to do and live this fantastic life. **Arlene Zanlunghi**, for your friendship, patience and understanding and **Michelle Wallace** for all your encouragement. **Lois Stewart**, culinary school would not have been the same without you and I am amazed that we are still close though it has been 32 years and 1,735 miles between us. **Chef Rex Leeson**, a Master Teaching Chef in school and **Chef John Alderson**, also a Master Teaching Chef, for believing in me and **Chef Glenn Dahl** (MTC) for pushing me.

My family. I believe that Chefs are born to be Chefs. The love of cooking and feeding people is deep in our soul. I began cooking with my brother. When we were little, I was 5 and he was 6 we would get up really early and clean the house (you can imagine how a 5 and 6 year old cleans) and make my parents breakfast in bed. Eggs, pancakes, whatever we could find to make. We would tell our parents **George and Norma La Vasseur**, that we got up and found the house clean and the "Pixies" left them breakfast with a note. I know that sounds darling, however, I was in my late 40"s before my mother confessed that those were some of the worst breakfasts they ever had. She said they would take a bite of what ever looked "safest to eat", tell us they had to get dressed and after we left, they would flush the breakfast down the toilet. They would then go hungry for the morning so we would not know.

I am grateful that I never knew. She said that after time, the breakfasts were actually good. Had I known from the beginning that the food was terrible, it would have demoralized my tender nature. I would have quit enjoying cooking. When I was a little older (still pulling up kitchen chairs to the stove so that I could reach the pots) I progressed to full dinners. Mom would let me pick a recipe from the "recipe file box" every week to try something new. My first cookbook was a gift from my brother, it was Julia Childs Menu Cookbook. What I learned from that book changed my world.

I am so grateful for my family and all the memories. Helping my grandmother, Anna La Vasseur, cook spurred my love for baking. I still enjoy canning because of her. Grandpa Calkins spaghetti sauce recipe was used in our restaurant and Grandma Calkins thanksgiving sage dressing will always be my favorite. **Aunt Lenora Sargent**, I am proud to be so much like you. **Mr. Buddy**, for your companionship while I wrote.

Introduction

I am Kathy Babbitt and as a classically trained chef, I thought living gluten free would be easy. I was wrong. I have been trying now for 11 years, and still get glutened from time to time. I have Hashimoto's disease which is an autoimmune disease. The disease causes your body to attack your thyroid when you eat foods that cause inflammation in your small intestines. The main culprit is gluten. It was years after being diagnosed with hypothyroidism that I found out the cause of my hypothyroidism was Hashimoto's. Consequently, that meant that all the symptoms that goes along with the digestive issues were misdiagnosed and mistreated. It is a story many of you know all too well.

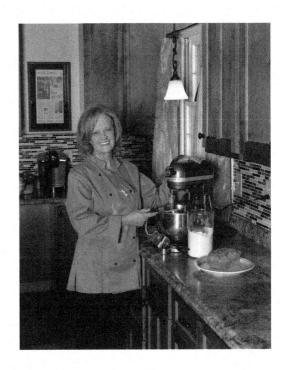

When I got the diagnosis of Hashimoto's it was life changing. I had been told by several doctors that I had it, but they did not do the blood test to confirm it so I did not know for sure. I was tested for Celiac disease and had all but 1 marker. The doctor told me again to cut out gluten. For years I was trying to not to eat gluten, but I was still not aware of everywhere it was. I was still having the "Lemon Butter" on my steak at Longhorn Steak House where I was a manager at that time. I was contaminating myself and not knowing it. Though I thought that I was eating correctly, I was still sick.

I was tired of being sick so I started doing research and was amazed at everywhere it is. I learned that not eating bread, cake, cookies, batter foods and gravy was not enough. I had been doing what I thought was enough. It was not. Living gluten free is difficult, very difficult. As a chef, I thought it would not be a problem to learn to cook without wheat, rye, and other gluten containing grains. However, over the years I have found it to be difficult to find recipes in books and on the internet that actually work. A great example is when I tried to make the eclairs that are in this book. I bought a book, recipe did not work…got on the internet and tried 4 different recipes from the internet and none worked. I was so frustrated! I regrouped and got out my old Professional Cooking Text Book and used it to make my own flour blend and used the classical technique to make them. Success on the first try!

I am now a lifestyle coach. I have a business called Gluten Intolerance Food Training (the G.I.F.T. Program from BABBITTS, INC). I am dedicated to helping people in a way that no one was there to help me. I teach them to cook gluten free (casein free… white sugar free… dairy free, etc.) in their homes, I help people learn to shop and to read ingredient panels. I help with cleaning out their kitchens if that is what they need. I hold classes in several locations in North Alabama on a variety of living gluten free challenges and solutions. I am a classical chef and pastry chef. I not only love to cook but love to teach cooking. It is very important that when I arrive at someone's home the recipe works, the first time! I might have to do product development for a week to get it right if it is something that is more difficult, but that is what I do. These recipes are the product of that work.

The recipes (formulas for the baking portion) have specific instructions and information as to why you have to do something a specific way. I did that so that you could understand the techniques and use them on other recipes when trying to convert a gluten recipe to a gluten free one. There is information on flours also. This is so you can experiment when you are ready and more confident.

Cooking is great fun. Play with your food! It is also a great family activity. My best childhood memories are cooking with grandparents, parents and friends. It amazes me how making something that was a favorite of someone important to you brings them home to you again. Many of these recipes were my grandmother, Anna La Vasseur. Some were my mothers, Norma La Vasseur, my other grandmother, Hazel Calkins, or my Aunt Lenora Sargent. I have no idea where they got them, I just know that they bring back great memories. Make great memories with your family. Food has brought people together for a very long time and will continue to do so.

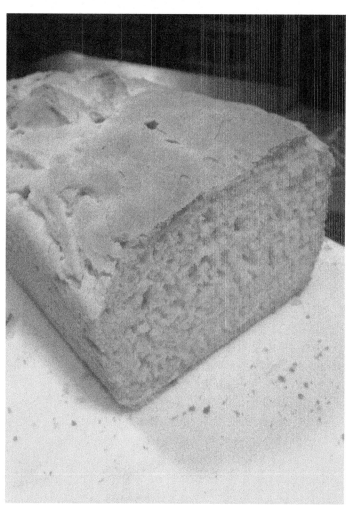

Most importantly though, when you or a family member has food intolerances or allergies, sometimes the only safe food is the food you make. So read through the book, check the ingredients on the packaged items you get for the recipes (ketchup, mustard and other foods can be potentially dangerous) and have fun!

Information

It's true that many of the food products typically eaten today contain gluten. Once you become familiar with navigating supermarket shelves, foods, and recipes for your diet, you'll find you can eat a variety of delicious foods without missing the glutinous ones. **Gluten free safe foods include fresh meats, fish, shellfish, fruits, vegetables, nuts and seeds, gluten-free grains, milk, and legumes.** Some of these foods may be unsafe if you have other food intolerances or allergies. The recipes in this book are primarily for eating gluten free though I do make notations for non-dairy substitutions when possible.

What is gluten?

Gluten is the generic name for certain types of proteins in grains like wheat, barley, rye, spelt, kamut, and triticale (a grain crossbred from wheat and rye). It is found in those grains and also wheat germ, wheat grass, wheat germ oil, graham flour, bulger, farina, couscous and semolina.

Oats and oat bran can be problematic as they may be cross contaminated with wheat. When using oats or oatmeal, choose brands that specify that they are gluten free.

When checking for gluten free on the label, remember that gluten free is considered by the FDA when the food is either naturally gluten free (like fresh fruits, vegetables, meats…) or has less than 20 ppm (parts per million) of gluten. However, for some people that is still too much. Some studies have shown that 1ppm or less of gluten is safe for celiac sufferers. Know what your tolerance is and work closely with your doctor so you are not unknowingly doing damage to your small intestines. This is especially true with Celiac disease, you can be doing damage to your small intestines and not have obvious symptoms. I am a fan of cooking your own food using fresh ingredients and avoiding prepackaged foods when possible. I understand that is not always possible with our busy lives, so please be careful!

From the FDA website:

Note: As of January 2014, "gluten-free" is defined as meaning the food either is inherently gluten-free or does not contain an ingredient that is: 1) a gluten-containing grain (e.g. spelt, wheat); 2) derived from a gluten-containing grain that has not been processed to remove gluten (e.g. wheat flour); or 3) derived from a gluten-containing grain that has been processed to remove gluten (e.g. wheat starch), if the use of that ingredient results in the presence of 20 parts per million (ppm) or more gluten in the food. To make the gluten-free claim on packaging, food manufacturers are required to test products and meet the FDA guidelines.

It is important to remember that wheat free does not mean gluten free. The FDA requires labeling of the 8 most common food allergies, of which wheat is one of. The top 8 allergen foods are milk, eggs, fish, shellfish, tree nuts, peanuts, wheat and soy beans. There is gluten in other grains, and so not listing wheat as an allergen alert does not make the food safe to eat.

Who does gluten sensitivity affect?

Estimates suggest 1 in 133 Americans suffers a reaction after ingesting gluten. Their reactions range from mild to very serious. Sadly not everyone who has a problem with gluten is aware of it. Here are a few of the conditions and symptoms:

Celiac Disease

Up to three million Americans are estimated to have celiac disease. This is the most serious of gluten-related conditions. Celiac disease is a genetic autoimmune disease that damages the small intestine and interferes with the absorption of nutrients from food when gluten is ingested. Some symptoms are gastrointestinal distress, chronic fatigue, osteoporosis, anemia, nutritional deficiencies and reproductive health issues. People with celiac disease must avoid gluten altogether to prevent destroying their small intestine or developing more serious diseases, including cancer.

Non-Celiac Gluten Sensitivity

Studies have determined that this is a real condition. The big difference between this and Celiac is that after you quit eating gluten and heal you gut, there is no more damage. That is only true if you do not eat gluten again because if you do you will be sick again. Different people have different tolerances, so again, work with you doctor and know your limitations. When you have a gluten intolerance and ingest it, you could experience digestive distress, skin irritation like eczema or hives, joint and muscle pain, fatigue, malabsorption of nutrients, headaches, or migraines.

Hashimoto's Thyroiditis

This is another autoimmune disease that is linked to gluten consumption. Hashimoto's disease causes your body to attack your thyroid. This leads to hypothyroidism and requires a lifetime of blood testing and medication. The list of symptoms are long and varied, and include weight gain, fatigue, joint and muscle pain, inability to get warm, difficulty getting pregnant, hair loss, depression, slow heart rate and gastrointestinal issues.

Allergies

People who have a wheat allergy, probably realize it. After ingesting wheat, you may quickly develop itchy and watery eyes, a runny nose, a skin rash, wheezing, or stomach discomfort. Eliminate wheat, and you'll likely eliminate your symptoms. You may be able to eat oats or rye gluten without a problem. Please note, wheat-free does not mean gluten-free on package labeling.

Lactose intolerance

It is not uncommon for people who have a problem with gluten to have a problem with the lactose in milk. Some also have a problem with casein which is a protein in dairy. I have made notations in the recipes when a substitute is okay. Different milks will have different tastes and textures. Experiment with the recipe and different milks to find what you like. For example, almond milk works better as a substitute in the white bread recipe than coconut milk…

There are many different gluten free flours to choose from and they all behave differently. When you are getting started, I would recommend either using Kathy's GFFM (Kathy's Gluten Free Flour Mix) that I have in this book or getting a good all-purpose gluten free flour mix. There are several on the market and others available on line that people recommend. Try the different blends and see which ones you and your family prefer. Before I made my own mix, I used King Arthur Flour © gluten free multi-purpose flour and their gluten free all-purpose baking mix. Should you not want to make your own blend, theirs will work in most recipes. It will not work in the eclairs, maple cake and the apple strudel, just to name a few recipes that my Kathy's GFFM is needed. Just remember that gluten free general purpose flours and gluten free baking mixes are NOT interchangeable. The General Purpose flours generally do not have a gum or leavening whereas the baking mixes usually do. Always read the ingredients on the package. Remember, different mixes work well for different applications. When the recipe is specific, use the flour that is specifically called for. It can get very expensive cooking with gluten free flours, the mix in this book can save you money.

Quinoa Flour- This flour is easy to digest and is loaded with great vitamins and minerals. It is also full of magnesium, protein, folate and zinc. It is rich with fiber. It has a nutty flavor and is great for muffins, banana bread, biscotti and shortcake.

Garbanzo Bean Flour. This is also known as Chick Pea Flour and is loaded with protein and fiber. It has a bean flavor that tastes great in savory dishes like meatloaf, falafel and burgers (though I prefer gluten free oatmeal for meatloaf and meat balls). It is also good for thickening stews and some soups.

Teff flour. This is the smallest grain in the world. It has a sweet and malty flavor once it is milled. It has high amounts of calcium and is a good source of iron. This flour is great for gluten free waffles, flat breads, anything chocolate and in cookies.

Buckwheat flour. This type of flour has an earthy flavor and contains high amounts of B vitamins and fiber. Use this flour to make pancakes, bar cookies, crepes, scones and quick breads.

Chia flour. This is derived from the ground seeds of the chia plant which is in the basil family. It is a dark flour and has a mildly nutty flavor. It can promote a healthy heart as it is high in omega 3 fatty acid. Because of the nutty flavor, it is great for brownies, muffins, sweet breads and crackers.

White Rice Flour. This is bland in taste and can come in several different textures. The finer the grind the less grittiness.

Another important factor with white rice flour is that it absorbs moisture slower, so letting the baked goods stand for a few minutes before baking will reduce grittiness.

Brown Rice Flour. This is packed with fiber and is made from different varieties like jasmine, long and short grain and basmati rice. There is a difference in how brown rice flour and white rice flour behave. They are not interchangeable.

Cornmeal Flour. Cornmeal flour is made from ground corn. You can use this to make polenta and other foods including corn bread. Always check that it is gluten free. Corn is another product that is subject to cross contamination in the transportation and manufacturing process.

Millet Flour. This is made by grinding millet seeds. It is golden and tastes nutty and sweet. It has lots of protein, B vitamins and lots of digestible fiber. I find that baked goods with millet flour tend to be flakier. It is excellent for pie crusts, but only as an addition to other flours, not a flour by itself.

Sorghum Flour. This flour has lots of antioxidants and has high amounts of fiber, iron and B vitamins. You usually use this flour with other flours and not normally by itself

Amaranth Flour. This comes from the seeds of amaranth plant. It is high in protein.

Arrowroot flour. This flour contains an easily digested starch from the roots of an arrowroot plant. It is used as a thickener in sauces and puddings. This flour works well with food that will need to be cooled and reheated as it does not break down as easily as corn starch. Use it to thicken gravy the same as you would if using wheat flour or cornstarch.

Tapioca Flour. It is mildly sweet and is used as an alternative to wheat flour. The starch is extracted from the cassava plant. It can be used in baked goods or used for thickening pie fillings, soups and sauces. Tapioca flour is similar in taste to wheat flour. It is sometimes sold as tapioca starch.

Coconut Flour. I love this flour. It is high in fiber. **It is made from coconut which is a nut, so those with a nut allergy cannot use this flour**. It makes great muffins and waffles.

Xanthan Gum. Gums are an important ingredient in gluten free baking. They add texture and allow the product to rise. Without them, your yeast or other leavening agent will rise, then the bubbles will just burst on the surface because there is no elasticity or structure to hold the air bubbles. Gluten normally provides elasticity to baked goods and without it, there is no elasticity and no real structure. Sometimes when you are having trouble getting bread to rise, try increasing the xanthan gum. The general rule is 1 teaspoon xanthan gum per 2 cups of flour. I increase this ratio though for some breads and pizza doughs to get more elasticity.

There are also other nut flours that can be wonderful to work with. Almond flour and pecan flour are just a couple of examples of other gluten free flours on the market.

As you can see, there is an extensive list of flours and it can be overwhelming to try to sort them all out. When starting out it can be very expensive to purchase all of these different flours. It is easier to start with a good blend, like the one I have in this book or getting a good mix that is on the market. Try the individual flours or make your own blend if you wish. Be careful to check the ingredients thoroughly. Some are rice flours and others are bean flours. Bean flours are good for some foods, but not necessarily for others. A bean cake for example might not be what you have in mind for a dinner party.

Safe ingredients to have in your kitchen

Whole foods and fresh foods are the safest gluten free foods to have in your home. Examples are chicken, fish, shellfish, beef, and pork, fresh vegetables some grains, fruits, legumes (check labels on canned varieties) nuts, seeds, honey, and maple syrup are all gluten free. The majority of your diet should contain these foods. They are all naturally gluten free as long as you do not add wheat breading or other ingredients that contaminate them. Some sauces, marinades and condiments (ketchup, mustard…) contain gluten so be careful to look for gluten free on the label.

Gluten free flour. This is flour that does not contain gluten at all. You can buy gluten free wheat flour (the gluten is processed out) but you can also substitute alternative flours that work really well. Different brands have different qualities and tastes so trying different flours with different recipes will help you find the flours you prefer.

Thickeners. Use cornstarch or arrowroot rather than a gluten containing flour when making sauces and gravies. Tapioca flour (sometimes called starch) works well also. They all have different attributes so use different thickeners for different applications.

Breading. The best I have found as a substitute for breading is Gluten Free Chex cereal. I crush it really fine. You can also use crushed potato chips, crushed corn tortilla chips or gluten free bread for breading.

Binders. There are several good binders. Xanthan gum, gelatin or guar gum all work great. Xanthan gum is my favorite. It is a little pricey, but you only use a small amount so it does last a really long time.

Snacks, Granola and Trail Mixes. Look for gluten free or make your own! I love making my own because I can make it with only the foods that I love and do not have to pick through a prepackaged mix for what I like. Granola can be made by using pure gluten free oats, nuts, seeds and other gluten free favorites. This is actually a great thing to have on hand for when you get hungry. Having snacks made up will make it easier for you to not give in to a gluten craving or other less than healthy snacks when you get hungry!

Plain popcorn (be careful of popcorn with flavorings as they can contain gluten), plain potato chips (check labels, some are not gluten free), plain corn chips, gluten free crackers and some granola bars are all safe to have for snacks. Remember to check labels though, some snacks available contain gluten ingredients.

Condiments. Always check the labels. Mustard, Ketchup, Peanut butter, Jelly and Jam, Soy Sauce and Worcestershire should all be fine. Some brands can also contain gluten. Strangely, some brands that are gluten free do not list that they are gluten free on the label. Call the number on the label or visit their website to find out if they are safe. Also, with some brands the ketchup is fine and the mustard is not… Again, check labels, do not assume that everything from a particular brand is safe. Also, do not share condiments with those eating gluten. Cross contamination is a real problem with sharing peanut butter, butters, jams, or any food that is spread on bread can be cross contaminated and you would not know it.

Spices. Spices are generally fine, but check the ingredients. It is not unusual for a spice blend to have flour as a thickener in it. I found this out the hard way with my favorite brand of chili seasoning…Some seasoning mixes use flour as an anti-caking agent, read the labels.

Grains. It is important to get enough grains in your diet. Several are safe. Amaranth, Buckwheat, Millet, Quinoa are all fine. Corn is also a grain as is rice.

Candies, Cookies and other sweets. Check labels. They may or may not contain gluten. A better option is fruit, but if you are really wanting sugary treats, make them. It is a great family activity and you control the ingredients! As a general statement, sugar is gluten free. Check labels though, anti-caking and thickening agents can be wheat…

Shopping

When shopping for your foods, it is critical that you read the labels. There are a lot more gluten free products on the market today then even a couple years ago. Some companies are now labeling their products that are gluten free. You can check the internet when it is not on the label and there are not specific ingredients that are concerning. Contact the manufacturer if you have any concerns and if there are any questions, choose another product. It is not worth the risk.

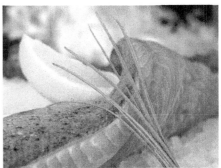

Try to shop the perimeter of the store. With a couple of exceptions, most grocery stores have the produce department, meat department and dairy departments on the perimeter of the store. Again, there are a couple of exceptions and I cannot speak to all stores in all areas, but the principal is the same. Fill your cart with fresh fruit, vegetables, nuts, meats, fish, and dairy (or dairy substitute if you are dairy free) and you will be on your way to safe, healthy eating.

When purchasing prepackaged foods, be careful to read the labels. Gluten free is not just "wheat free". Wheat is one of the top allergens so companies have to list it. The FDA requires all top allergens to be listed on the label. That covers dairy, eggs, fish, shellfish, soy, wheat, nuts and peanuts. Gluten is in other grains also. It is not only in wheat (wheat germ, wheat grass, wheat germ oil), it is also in rye, barley, kamut, spelt, triticale, graham flour, malt, bulger, and farina (cream of wheat cereal), couscous and semolina. It can be in oats due to cross contamination, so be careful to only use gluten free oats.

The Gluten Free Social Life

Being gluten free can be difficult. With so much of our diet involving enriched flour, it is challenging for us and those that are hosting us to provide food that will not make us sick. When dining out and at a dinner party, pre planning is key.

When dining out, look online for menus, especially gluten free. Ask for the chef or manager and let them know what your dietary restrictions are. Look for ingredients on the menu that are fresh. Order whole muscle meat, fish, seafood and chicken, vegetables and fruits are naturally gluten free. The problem can be how it is prepared. Ask questions and avoid batters, seasonings, sauces and items cooked with other contaminated items, such as deep fried foods. Choose restaurants that are traditionally whole foods and made to order. That allows greater flexibility in the kitchen for the cooks to omit items you cannot have.

When at a dinner party, Pre planning will make all the difference. It is smart to pack something to eat, eat before you go or bring an item for all to share if going to someone's home for dinner. Always ask first though. You can package it as a hostess gift if you are not comfortable asking, just make sure it is just an appetizer and not entrée or dessert. Going to dinner not terribly hungry will help you make smart choices and not become irritable when there is little to eat.

Always show appreciation and be graceful when saying "no thank you"

There will be people who are supportive and really try to help you. There will be others who are disagreeable and think that you are just difficult. Be kind to both. Those who are really trying, reading recipes, and are so proud of their accomplishment, may still not understand all of the complexities and cross contamination problems. Still be kind.

There are times when you are out and someone offers you something you have to refuse, be gracious and just say "no, thanks."

Cross Contamination.

This is of particular concern in homes where people are eating gluten containing foods and someone is gluten free. When equipment and utensils are shared, gluten can contaminate the gluten free food, making someone sick. Be careful to not share dish cloths and sponges, cutting boards, and any plastic utensils. Gluten is very sticky and does not die at high temperatures. It can stick to a cutting board and then when used for preparing food for the non-gluten eater, it can contaminate it. Remember the FDA says that 20 ppm is safe. That is .002%, and some studies, as stated earlier, maintain that is still too much. One crumb transferred on the same knife used on wheat toast and then gluten free toast is enough to make someone sick for example.

Cross contamination can occur when sharing condiments such as mustard, mayonnaise and jam's. This is as simple as using the same knife in the peanut butter to make a gluten free sandwich and a gluten sandwich. It can happen innocently and then someone gets sick and you do not know why. When accidents happen in our home, we put a big black X on the container so I know I cannot use it. A good solution is to either have separate condiments for gluten eaters and non-gluten eaters or use squeeze bottles to avoid any possible cross contamination.

There is a lot of information on the internet about making your home safe when some are eating gluten and some are not. When children are involved, there is a greater need to be particularly careful. Keep foods that can make them sick in a separate cupboard, out of reach. Talk to your health care professional and visit our website at www.lovinglivingglutenfree. com or www.thebabbitts.net to learn more about cross contamination.

Gluten free can be delicious! When using the recipes in this book, please read the entire recipe before beginning. Also, some of the steps are specific as are some of the ingredients. This is very important. When a substitution is okay, I have noted it, otherwise, please use the specified ingredient. Also, some of the steps may seem different then when making a similar food with wheat flour. The gluten free flours behave differently, so there are steps that you do that will make the recipe work. Omitting some of the steps could possibly change to success of the recipe.

When using gluten free flours, the absorption of moisture is different than when using traditional wheat flours. When the finished product is gritty, it can because the flour has not absorbed the required moisture to soften the flour. In most of my recipes (formulas for baked goods) one of the steps is to let the item rest. In gluten baking that can be required to let the gluten rest. In gluten free baking, it is to allow the flours to absorb the moisture. This is especially important with white rice flour. When there is a leavening used, like baking powder or baking soda, the resting time is as short as possible. Baking soda and baking powder are activated by moisture, so the item will begin to rise too quickly if the resting time is too long.

When making these items, please note that not only the flours make a difference, but also changing the oils will change the recipe. I have noted when other oils can be used. When coconut oil is used, do not try to remove the item from the pan for at least 10 minutes as it can stick. You could use coconut oil for frying, however, the smoke point for coconut oil is 350°F which is the same as butter, and sesame oil. This means that you have to be careful when using this oil that it does not get too hot and start to smoke. Using peanut oil (if no peanut allergy) or safflower oil works great for the deep frying in the donut recipe.

I believe it is important to know the smoke point temperatures for oils. Temperature smoke points for oils are: Extra virgin olive oil is 325°F which makes it a bad choice for sautéing, though many do use it to sauté, vegetable shorting is 360°F and Vegetable oil is 400°F. Light refined olive oil has a smoke point of 465°F making it a great choice for sautéing. Safflower oil is great for high temperatures, it is good to 450°F. Why does this matter? The smoke point is where the oil is breaking down and releasing free radicals and the food will taste scorched or burnt. This is the point where your kitchen become stinky and someone says "I think something is burning" or "I hear the dinner bell" as the smoke detector is going off. Of greater concern though is that smoking oil is signaling that it is getting to the point that the oil can catch fire. Frying with an oil that has a low smoke point is fine as long as it is fresh and you are very careful about the temperature you are using it at. However, if your oil starts to smoke, turn off the heat and let it cool slightly. Anytime you are deep frying, do not leave the food unattended and when children are present, use the back burners and stay at the fryer (stove). Avoid accidents! Most oils have the smoke point stated on the label. Try to use the right oil for the cooking that you are doing.

Most of the formulas and recipes are suitable for alternative sugars. None of these recipes call for sugar substitutes. There is a lot of interesting research on the use of sugar substitutes. That is not my area of expertise so please check with your doctor before using them. Using coconut sugar for the baked goods is fine, but the color will change. It is a brown sugar and is coarser than cane white or brown sugar. The eclairs pictured in this book has pastry cream made with coconut sugar and the color is light tan not bright yellow for example. The taste is really good though and if your concern is glycemic index, coconut sugar is a great choice (again, it is a nut though, so those with nut allergies cannot use coconut sugar). Use the liquid from the recipe to soften the coconut sugar. Add the sugar to the liquid and after the sugar has softened for about 5 minutes, stir it and add it to the other ingredients. This extra step will result in a smoother texture to the finished product. This is especially true for cookies, muffins, breads and cakes.

Gluten free breads can take longer to rise, be patient and plan early…Also, should you have trouble getting the bread to rise, try increasing the xanthan gum, not the yeast. Because you do not have gluten, if there is not enough xanthan gum, the structure of the bread is too weak and cannot hold the bread when it is rising.

Lastly, all of the recipes in this book use my flour blend unless otherwise stated. There are a lot of flour blends out there now, so should you have one that you like, by all means try it in these recipes. I use my blend because I find that with simple adjustments or additions (millet flour, sorghum flour, etc.…) it works no matter what I need.

When mixing, the times specified have to do with all the ingredients mixing together properly. You cannot over mix gluten free flours, but you can incorporate in too much air for some items. The mixing times for cookies with standard gluten flours has to do with developing the gluten, giving the mix structure. An over mixed cookie with gluten flour will result in a tough cookie for example. That does not apply to gluten free baking as there is not any gluten to over develop.

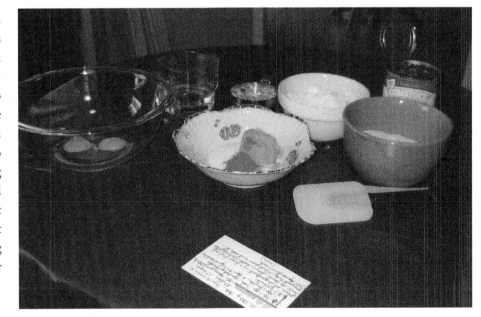

KATHY'S GLUTEN FREE FLOUR MIX (KATHY'S GFFM)

Here is my Gluten Free Flour Mixture. I use this when I bake and any recipes that make reference to my mix are referring to this. I do also mention other flours that work well that are readily available in your local grocery store.

2 pounds white rice flour
1 pound brown rice flour
2 pounds corn starch (check that it is gluten free)

Mix in a very large bowl with a whisk and then sift at least 2 times into another large bowl. You can make less, just keep the ratios correct.

The ratios are by weight. The weight of these flours are not the same. So an example of a smaller batch is:

1 cups white rice flour
½ cup + 2 tablespoons brown rice flour
1 cups + 2 tablespoon cornstarch
This would make 2 ¾ cup flour

You can substitute tapioca flour for the corn starch if you have a problem with corn starch. Most of the recipes will work fine with that adjustment.

Breakfast Foods

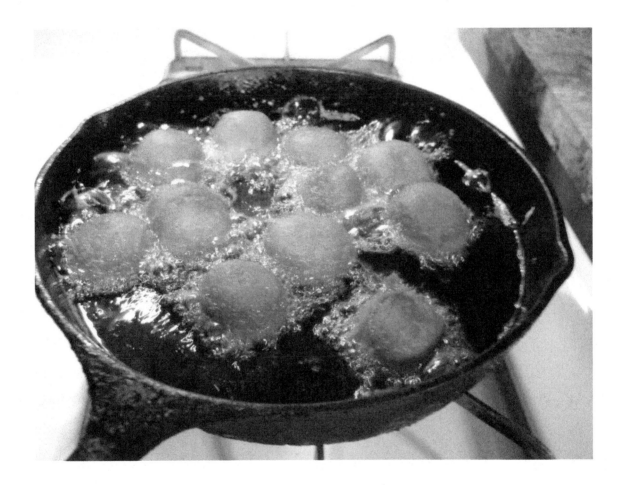

Donuts

One of the things that I hear that people miss the most is donuts. These are fantastic "cake" donuts, like a sour cream donut. I do find that making a "donut whole" cooks better. You can use a donut pan and bake them if you prefer.

2 ⅔ cup Kathy's GFFM page 18
1 teaspoon baking soda
1 teaspoon baking powder
1 ½ teaspoon xanthan gum
¼ cup butter
¼ cup coconut oil (or vegetable oil)
½ cup sugar
⅓ cup brown sugar (coconut sugar works well)
2 large eggs
1 teaspoon vanilla extract
½ teaspoon cinnamon
1 cup milk
Oil for frying

With a wire whisk mix the flour blend, baking soda, baking powder and xanthan gum in a bowl and set aside

In the bowl of a stand mixer, beat together the butter, oil and sugars until smooth. Add the eggs, one at a time and beat until well combined.

Stir the vanilla and cinnamon into the milk

Stir in the flour mixture into the butter mixture alternately with the milk mixture. Begin and end with the flour mixture. Mix well making sure everything is combined.

Let stand for 10 minutes.

Heat oil to 350°F

Drop the dough into hot oil using a teaspoon or small scoop. Fry until golden and then flip in the oil using either a wooden spoon or long wooden skewers. Do not use plastic, it can melt due to the heat of the oil. Flip as often as needed to achieve a nice golden brown donut. When done, remove from oil and strain on paper towels to absorb excess oil.

Top with cinnamon sugar, powdered sugar or glaze. When using powdered sugar or cinnamon sugar, the sugar will stick when the donuts are still warm. The maple glaze that is used on the maple pound cake is perfect for the donuts!

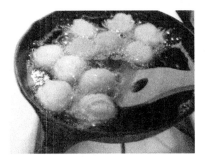 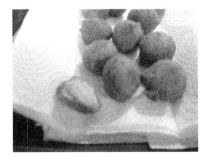 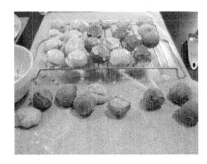

Gluten Free Danish

The formula and steps to make the Danish are on the next 4 pages. Though there are a lot of steps, it is worth the effort. The dough freezes as does the finished product for use in the future. When freezing the dough, let it thaw before using. You will still want it to be cold, just not frozen.

¼ cup white sugar (organic evaporated cane juice sugar is fine)
½ cup water, room temperature
2 teaspoons yeast

1 ¾ cups Kathy's GFFM page 18
½ cup almond flour
½ cup tapioca starch
¼ cup millet flour
1 tablespoon xanthan gum
½ teaspoon salt
½ teaspoon cardamom if desired
1 ¾ sticks butter, cold and cut into 1 tablespoon chunks*

1 egg
1 egg yolk

Mix the yeast and water and sugar and set aside to soften.

Combine the flours, starch, xanthan gum, salt and cardamom in the bowl of a stand mixer and whisk to combine.

Cut in the butter into the flour mixture with a pastry knife until it resembles small to medium size peas. Some of the flour will not be cut in. That is okay. It should be a powdery mix. Do not over process.

When the yeast becomes foamy, add the egg and the egg yolk to the yeast mixture and mix. Then add to the flour mixture.

Using a stand mixer, mix on medium until a smooth dough forms. Beat on medium for an additional 5 minutes. You may add small amounts of additional flour if necessary, the dough should be somewhat sticky, but hold its shape and not stick to the side of the bowl. The dough will seem really greasy but it is not greasy when done baking.

Form into a ball and wrap in plastic wrap. Refrigerate for 2 hours to overnight before beginning the turns.

To begin turns, roll the dough out in a rectangle; fold the dough onto itself in thirds, like folding a letter. Roll out into a rectangle again about ¼ to ⅛ inch thick. Repeat this process 3 times. Repeat this process 3 times. This process is easiest if you roll the pastry on a large size (full sheet pan) parchment with a piece of plastic wrap on top. Dust the parchment with gluten free flour or corn starch to help prevent sticking while you are doing the turns.

This method does not require folding in a butter/flour layer that is normally done when you make Danish. This was not an accidental omission. The butter is cut into the dough. The flours in the dough are not strong enough to fold in a butter layer without tearing the dough. When the dough tears, the butter leaks out.

*Use a gluten free dairy free butter spread if making dairy free. Use ¾ cup if using the spread or 1 ½ sticks of gluten free dairy free butter spread if you have sticks.

Fillings for Danish

Cinnamon sugar with butter:

½ stick butter, softened
3 tablespoons white or brown sugar
1 tablespoon cinnamon
Spread the butter over the pastry. Sprinkle with the cinnamon sugar. Roll jelly roll style and slice in about 1 ½ to 2 inch slices. Bake on a parchment lined baking sheet for 15-20 minutes.

Almond filling:

½ pound almond paste
½ cup white sugar (you can use organic or coconut sugar if you wish)
½ cup butter
¼ cup Kathy's GFFM page 18
1 egg
Using the paddle attachment on a stand mixer, mix almond paste and sugar at low speed until mixed. Mix in the butter and flour. Beat in egg and mix until smooth.

Roll out the dough and cut into about 6 inch squares. Place the filling in the center of the dough and fold over. Seal the edge with an egg wash (1 egg and ½ cup milk or milk substitute) and then cut the dough in 3 "slices" along the fold, not the seam. Turn the dough out slightly to make "bear paws" see picture on page 30.

Chocolate filling

¼ cup sugar (you can use organic or coconut sugar if you wish)
⅛ cup cocoa
1 teaspoon vanilla
½ cup biscuit crumbs, cake crumbs or cookie crumbs (from gluten free biscuits, cookie or cakes)
1 tablespoon butter

Mix all ingredients well. Roll out the dough and cut into about 4" squares. Place the filling in the center of the square and bring 2 opposite corners into the center over the filling and seal the tips together with egg wash.

Preheat the oven to 400°F

Separate the dough into halves and keep one refrigerated while working with the other. Cold dough works best. Prepare baking sheets with parchment unless they are non-stick.

Dust a clean counter surface, rolling matt, or parchment with gluten free flour mix or corn starch and roll into a square. The dough should be about ¼ to 1/8 inch thick. Cut into squares about 4-6 inches on each side. Fill with your choice of filling and fold into your desired shape. For pinwheels, cut in from the 4 corners diagonally into the center, not cutting the center, and put a dollop of filling in the center. Then fold the left corner of each cut into the center and brush with egg wash. Transfer to a non-stick cookie sheet. The dough can be fragile so be careful transferring to a cookie sheet. A wide pancake turner or bench knife works best. Sometimes I transfer the squares to the cookie sheet and then form my shapes from there. Cover and let rest for about 30 -45 minutes in a warm place to rise. Top with egg wash before baking if you desire to assist in browning (1 egg beaten and 1 cup milk or almond milk and brushed on top of the pastry). Bake in preheated oven at 400°F. They should take 10-12 minutes to bake depending on size. Larger, thicker pastries will take longer to bake.

Bear paws

Pinwheels

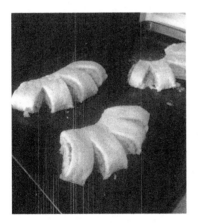
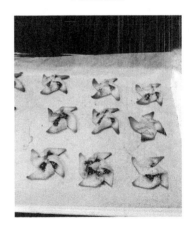

Gluten Free Biscuits

½ cup butter (coconut oil, solid, do not melt, or GFCF substitute if you need it to be dairy free)
2 cups Kathy's GFFM page 18
1 teaspoon xanthan gum
1 teaspoon baking soda
1/3 cup butter milk (use almond milk if you need it to be dairy free.)*
2 large eggs

Preheat the oven to 400°F.

Mix the flour, xanthan gum and baking soda in a bowl. With a pastry knife, cut the butter into the flour mix until small pea shaped dough clumps form.

With a wire whisk (by hand) mix the milk and the large eggs. Then with a wooden spoon, mix the milk and eggs into the baking mix/butter mixture.

Lightly dust your cleaned work surface with corn starch and turn the dough out onto the work surface.

Fold the dough over onto itself 4 times and then roll out to about ¾ to 1 inch thick. Cut dough with a 2 ½ inch round cutter and place onto a non stick cookie sheet approximately 1 inch apart. You can also use parchment lined cookie sheet. Carefully rework the scraps by stacking them and pressing together and rolling out to the same thickness, cutting them into biscuits and place them on the baking pan also.

Bake the biscuits for about 14 to 18 minutes until they're light golden brown. You can egg wash them if you desire greater glossiness and browning. Remove them from the oven and let them rest for about 10 minutes. They are best served warm.

* You can also use sour milk in place of butter milk. When you do not have either, add 1 teaspoon lemon juice to milk or almond milk and let sit for about 5 minutes.

Gluten Free French Toast

Gluten Free Bread*

For every 2 slices of bread cooked you will need
1 egg
2 tablespoons milk (or almond milk)
Splash of gluten free vanilla
Cinnamon and powdered sugar.

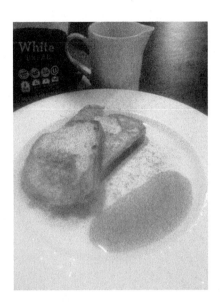

Turn on a skillet to begin heating it. Spray with gluten free pan coating before putting the French toast on the skillet.

Whisk the egg, milk and vanilla in a flat bowl (a pie plate works best)

Soak the bread, first one side than the other and then transfer to the skillet. Cook on a hot skillet that has been sprayed with gluten free pan coating.

Cook until browned and then flip to other side and cook until done.

Dust with cinnamon and powdered sugar and serve warm with jam or syrup as you prefer.

*I prefer kinikinnick foods© Gluten Free white bread for this recipe.

Breads

There is life after gluten.

Store breads for a short time in the refrigerator, for longer storage, slice and store in the freezer. Gluten free breads stale quickly. They are best enjoyed the day baked.

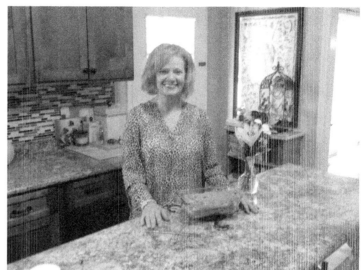

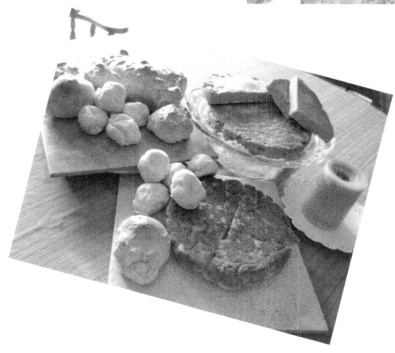

Nut Bread

I love this bread!

2 ½ cups Kathy's GFFM page 18
1 ½ teaspoon xanthan gum
1 teaspoon salt
3 tablespoons coconut oil, melted
1 cup white sugar
3 ½ teaspoons baking powder
1 ¼ cup milk
1 egg
1 cup chopped nuts (I prefer walnuts)
2 teaspoons grated orange zest or 1 tablespoon orange juice

Preheat oven to 350

Grease and flour a 9x5x3 inch loaf pan or small demi loaf pans if you prefer.

Mix the flour, xanthan gum, baking powder and salt in a bowl and whisk to combine.

Mix the oil and sugar in the bowl of a stand mixer and mix well. Add the egg to the milk and then add to the oil and sugar mixture.

Add the dry ingredients to the oil, sugar mixture in the mixing bowl mix on low to incorporate all ingredients well and then beat on medium speed for 2 minutes.

Clean bowl and beaters during mixing process as necessary.

Pour into pans, bake 55 to 65 minutes until a wooden tester inserted in the center comes out clean. Demi loaf pans will cook in about 20-30 minutes until a wooden tester comes out clean. Let cool in pan for 10 minutes and then loosen from side of pan, turn out of pan to finish cooling.

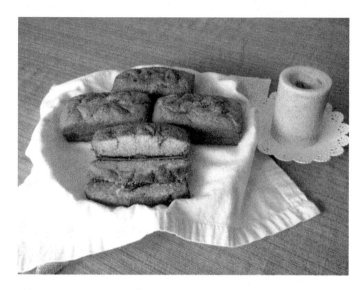

Cinnamon Bread

Filling

3 tablespoons white sugar (coconut sugar works well too)
1 tablespoon ground cinnamon

For the batter

2 cups Kathy's GFFM page 18
1 teaspoon baking powder
1 teaspoon baking soda
1 teaspoon xanthan gum
¼ teaspoon salt
1 stick unsalted butter softened
1 cup white sugar (organic or coconut sugar works great also)
2 large eggs
1 teaspoon vanilla
1 cup buttermilk*
Heat oven to 350°F and grease a 9x5x3" loaf pan or demi pans.

Mix the milk and lemon juice if not using buttermilk. (See note at the bottom of the page.)

Mix the filling: Mix the sugar and cinnamon in a small bowl and set aside.

Make the batter: In a medium bowl, mix the flour, baking powder, baking soda, xanthan gum and salt and mix well.

In a mixing bowl of a stand mixer, cream the butter and sugar until light and fluffy. Add the eggs, one at a time and beat well after each addition. Add the vanilla and mix well. Scrape down the sides of the bowl and beater as necessary.

Alternately add the flour mixture and the buttermilk to the butter mixture. Start and end with the flour mixture stirring well between each addition. Continue to blend until all ingredients are completely blended in.

Spoon first layer of batter into pan (1/2 the batter for one pan and 1/8 batter if using 4 demi pans), sprinkle filling over batter and then cover with batter and top with the filling.

Bake until golden brown and a wooden tester inserted in the center comes out clean. A full loaf takes 50-60 minutes and 20-30 for demi loaves.

Remove from the pan from the oven and immediately remove the bread from the pan. Let cool on the wire rack

*You can use milk or Almond Milk. Use Almond milk if you want to make this casein free. You will need to add1 teaspoon lemon to sour the milk (either used) if not using buttermilk. You will need to let it stand for about 5 minutes, so do this step first.

Pretzel Bread

Oh my... spread with cream cheese instead of butter and it is soft pretzel time!

3 cups Kathy's GFFM page 18
¼ cup tapioca flour
2 ½ teaspoon xanthan gum
1 tablespoon instant yeast
¼ teaspoon cream of tarter
½ teaspoon baking soda
1 tablespoon packed brown sugar
1 teaspoon salt
1 teaspoon apple cider vinegar
2 tablespoons unsalted butter, softened
1 egg
1 ½ cup buttermilk*

Grease the bottom of a 9X3 loaf pan up the side about 1".

Add the yeast to the buttermilk and set aside to activate the yeast.

In the bowl of a stand mixer, mix the flours, xanthan gum, cream of tartar, baking soda, brown sugar and salt. Mix with a wire whisk to combine all ingredients well.

Add the vinegar, butter and eggs to the flour mixture and with the mixer on low, stir to combine. Add the yeast and buttermilk and stir on low until all ingredients are incorporated. Turn the mixer to medium and mix for 3 minutes. Stop the mixer and scrape the sides as needed.

The dough will be damp, but will pull from the sides of the bowl. Add more Kathy's GFFM flour if needed by small amounts so that the dough does form a ball, but it will be moist.

Form the dough with your hands into the pan shape and put it in the prepared pan to rise. Leave the dough in a warm location to rise, about 1 hour. It should almost double in size.

Preheat the oven to 375°F while the dough is rising.

Bake the dough in the oven for 50-60 minutes until done. The bread should reach an internal of 190-200°F.

You can egg was the dough to help with browning if you wish.

Egg Wash: 1 egg and ½ cup milk, whisk to combine well and brush on top of the bread to help in browning.

Serve warm.

*You can substitute sour milk for buttermilk. When you do not have either, mix 1 teaspoon lemon juice into the milk and let stand for 5 minutes to sour.

Gluten Free Corn Bread

Corn bread is something that I missed terribly. This one is moist, flavorful and easy to make. It can be made dairy free easily using coconut milk. It is also fantastic with kefir. I like to use coconut sugar in this recipe. Coconut sugar and coconut milk together does change it the recipe. It is still good, but does not taste like traditional corn bread.

1 cup Kathy's GFFM page 18
1 cup yellow cornmeal
1 cup millet flour
1 tablespoon xanthan gum
1 tablespoon baking powder
¾ teaspoons salt
½ teaspoon baking soda
¼ cup melted butter (or melted coconut oil for dairy free)
½ cup white sugar (or coconut sugar if you prefer)
1 ½ cup buttermilk (or kefir, coconut milk also works in this recipe if you are dairy free)
3 large eggs

Preheat oven to 375

Lightly grease the bottom and sides of a 9x9 baking pan or a 9x5x3 loaf pan.

Whisk together the flours, xanthan gum, baking powder, salt and baking soda.

In a separate bowl whisk together the melted butter, sugar, milk and eggs until smooth.

Add the wet ingredients to the dry ingredients. Mix until smooth.

Pour the batter into the prepared pan and let stand for 10 minutes uncovered.

Bake for 30-40 minutes for the 9x9 pan and about 55 minutes for a loaf pan, until the bread is golden brown. The internal temperature has to be 190°F. Use a thermometer, as this is about 3-5 minutes past when inserting a toothpick in the center will come out clean. Check the temperature in the center of the cornbread and any other location that appears to be less brown to be sure the temperature is correct.

Cool for at least 5 minutes before turning out of the pan and cutting. Serve warm. This recipe freezes beautifully and is excellent for making cornbread dressing!

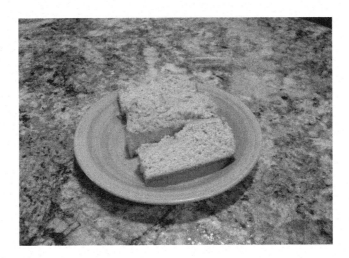

Gluten Free White Bread

This bread can be made dairy free also.

2 cups Kathy's GFFM page 18
2 teaspoons xanthan gum
1 teaspoon salt
½ cup water
½ cup milk (almond milk for dairy free bread)
2 ¼ teaspoons active dry yeast (1 package)
3 tablespoons honey
¼ cup Kathy's GFFM page 18 (this in addition to the flour listed above.)
2 eggs
2 tablespoons butter or Gluten Free Dairy Free butter substitute
1 tablespoon cider vinegar

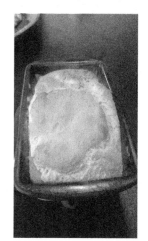

Prepare 1 9x5x3" bread pan. I recommend greasing the bottom and about ½ inch up the side. This allows the bread to rise and not fall when cooling. It will need to be loosened with a knife when cooled (after about 10 minutes) before turning out of the pan or it will stick.

Measure the dry ingredients a bowl and using a wire whisk mix the ingredients to blend.

Place the milk and water in a bowl (or pan if warming on the stove) and heat to 100 degrees*. Add the yeast, honey and the additional ¼ cup of gluten free flour blend. Let stand until foamy.

Mix the eggs, butter and cider in the bowl of a stand mixer with the paddle attachment. The butter will be chunky, that is alright.

On low speed add half the dry ingredients to the egg mixture and mix until blended, add half the liquid yeast ingredients, mix until thoroughly incorporated and then add the remaining dry and then the remaining wet ingredients.

When all ingredients are incorporated and mixed in, turn the mixer to medium speed and beat for 4 minutes. The dough will look like cake batter.

Preheat the oven to 375°F

Spoon into the pan and set aside to rise about 50 minutes. Gluten free breads can take longer to rise especially if not in a warm place. Do not be discouraged if it has not doubled in size in 50 minutes. Give it more time or cook when risen and additional ½ in size for a denser bread.

Bake in oven for 40-55 minutes until the bread reaches an internal temperature of 200 degrees. This bread browns beautifully, you can also use an egg wash to give it a glossy look. Egg wash is made with 1 egg whisked with ½ cup milk or almond milk.

Cool for 10 minutes before turning out the bread to cool.

*Yeast begins to die at 120°F and completely dies at 140°F. It is very important that you take the temperature of the liquid with a thermometer.

Gluten Free Rolls, Hamburger Buns or Hot Dog Buns.

The previous recipe with the following adjustment:

1 ½ cup Kathy's GFFM page 18
½ cup potato starch

All the remaining ingredients and steps apply until the panning

Instead of panning in a bread pan, use a portion scoop to either make rolls or burger buns. The size of the scoop makes the difference. A 2 ounce scoop to make rolls and a 4 ounce scoop to make hamburger buns. Use a spoon to make a long bun for a hot dog bun. Pan on a cookie sheet lined with parchment.

Leave in a warm area to raise and then bake @ 375°F until golden brown. Times will vary depending on the size of the rolls.

Pita/Naan Bread

½ cup water heated to 100°F1 tablespoon raw honey
2 teaspoons instant dry yeast
½ cup milk (use Almond Milk for dairy free)
1 tablespoon cider vinegar
2 cups Bob's Red Mill Pizza Crust Flour Mix©
2 tablespoons psyllium husk
½ teaspoon xanthan gum
1 ½ teaspoon salt
¼ teaspoon baking powder
¼ cup extra virgin olive oil
2 large eggs beaten

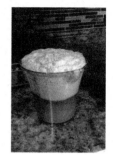

Mix the water, honey and yeast in a bowl and set aside to activate the yeast and create a foam.

Mix the milk and cider vinegar and set aside to sour.

Mix the pizza flour, psyllium husk, xanthan gum, salt and baking powder and whisk to combine.

When the yeast mixture has created a foam, whisk in the olive oil and beaten eggs

Pour the liquid over the dry mixture and stir to combine.

Add the milk mixture and stir to combine.

Let the dough rest for 20 minutes.

Turn a skillet on to heat

Dust the counter with some pizza flour or cornstarch and turn the dough out. Separate into 6-8 balls

Dust the top of the dough with some more pizza flour or cornstarch and carefully roll and pat the dough flat

Transfer to a skillet and using the spatula carefully flatten the bread in the skillet until it is about 1/3 inches thick.

Cook for about 2 minutes on each side turning as necessary and watch carefully so they do not burn.

Serve warm or cool. You can cut in half and then carefully cut into the center of the bread and open a pocket for pita bread.

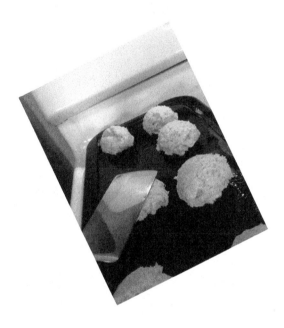

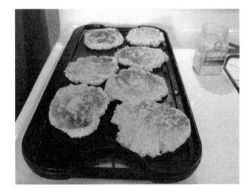

Focaccia Bread

1 ½ cup Kathy's GFFM page 18
½ cup amaranth flour
¼ cup potato starch
1 teaspoon baking powder
1 ¼ teaspoon salt
1 ½ teaspoon xanthan gum
1 tablespoon sugar
2 ¼ teaspoon yeast
1 ½ cup milk
3 tablespoons olive oil
1 tablespoon olive oil (in addition to amount above)
½ teaspoon Italian seasoning
Pinch of garlic salt and a pinch of cracked black pepper
Preheat oven to 350°F

Grease or use pan spray on the bottom of a 9" cake pan.

Heat milk to 100°F. Add the sugar and 3 tablespoons olive oil and yeast and mix. Set aside to activate the yeast and get foamy.

Mix the flours, baking powder, salt and xanthan gum in the bowl of a stand mixer with a wire whisk.

When the yeast is foamy, mix into the dry mixture with a stand mixer. When all liquid is incorporated, beat on medium for 2 minutes.

Let stand while preparing the pan.

Pour 1 tablespoon in the center of a 9" round cake pan and swirl to coat the pan. The entire pan does not have to be covered with olive oil. Sprinkle the seasonings over the olive oil. Spoon the batter over the olive oil and place in a warm place to rise.

Bake when doubled in size for about 30 minutes until done. It will not be browned on the top when done. The internal temperature should be 200°F.

When done, remove from the oven and let stand for 10 minutes before removing from pan. Flip the bread out of the pan after 10 minutes onto a serving platter. This bread is excellent warm!

You can also use this recipe to make pita bread. Let the dough stand for 30 minutes covered. Heat a skillet and scoop the dough into the skillet and press down with a metal pancake turner dipped in olive oil to flatten. Turn frequently to prevent burning. Cool. They do not make a "pocket" but you can cut a pocket in them or use it as a wrap for sandwiches.

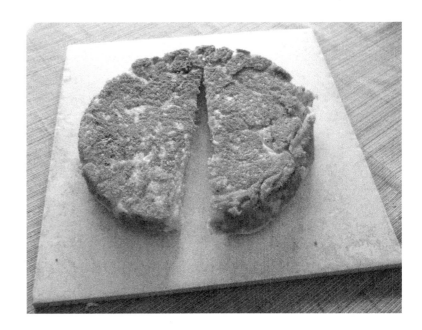

Falafel Bread

1 1/2 cup milk (or almond milk for dairy free) warm to 100 degrees

2 tablespoons white sugar (coconut sugar or organic sugar)

3 tablespoons olive oil

4 teaspoons active dry yeast (1 tablespoon + 1 teaspoon)

2 1/2 cups Bobs Red Mill All Purpose Baking Flour© (or a garbanzo bean flour)

3/4 cup cornstarch

1/2 cup white rice flour

1/4 cup psyllium husk

1/4 cup amaranth flour

1 tablespoon xanthan gum

2 teaspoons cumin (less might be better if you do not prefer cumin, it is very flavorful!)

1 1/2 teaspoons kosher or sea salt

2 teaspoons dried chives

2 large eggs lightly beaten

1 teaspoon apple cider vinegar

16 ounce can garbanzo beans rinsed drained and chopped (I used a pastry knife)

Mix the warm milk, sugar and olive oil, add the yeast and stir lightly. Set the yeast aside to foam (some call it a sponge).

Mix the flours, psyllium husk, xanthan gum, cumin, salt and chives in the bowl of a stand mixer and whisk to combine ingredients well. Add the yeast mixture and turn the mixer on low. Add the eggs and apple cider vinegar. Mix to combine then turn the mixer to medium speed and mix for 4 minutes. Stir in the chopped chick peas.

Form into 4 balls (or one large loaf, 2 loaves, or rolls, whatever you prefer) with wet hands and place on a prepared cookie sheet (2 loaves per sheet to allow room for rising) and put in a warm place to rise until double in size. Preheat oven to 375°F

Bake in 375°F oven for approximately 40 minutes (depending on what size you are cooking, larger loaves will take longer than small loaves and rolls) until browned and an internal temperature of 190°-200°F is reached.

Sweet Potato Bread

1 cup Kathy's GFFM page 18
½ cup millet flour
2 teaspoons baking powder
1 teaspoon xanthan gum
¼ teaspoon salt
1 teaspoon ground nutmeg
½ teaspoon ground cinnamon
1 cup white sugar (or coconut sugar)
2 eggs, beaten
½ cup melted coconut oil (or vegetable oil)
2 tablespoon milk
1 cup cooked mashed sweet potato
1 cup chopped pecans
½ cup raisins

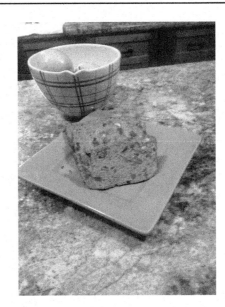

Preheat oven to 325°F, Grease an 8x5x" loaf pan.

Stir dry ingredients in the bowl of a stand mixer with a whisk.

Combine sugar, eggs, oil and milk. When using coconut sugar, let stand 5 minutes to soften the coconut sugar. I usually use coconut sugar when making this bread.

Mix the wet ingredients into the dry on low speed. Mix until ingredients are incorporated.

Fold in the sweet potatoes, pecans and raisins, and mix until well combined.

Pour into the prepared pan. Bake 70 minutes until a tester comes out clean when inserted into the center. This bread should cook to an internal temperature of 190 to 200°F. Cool for 15 minutes in the pan before turning out to cool.

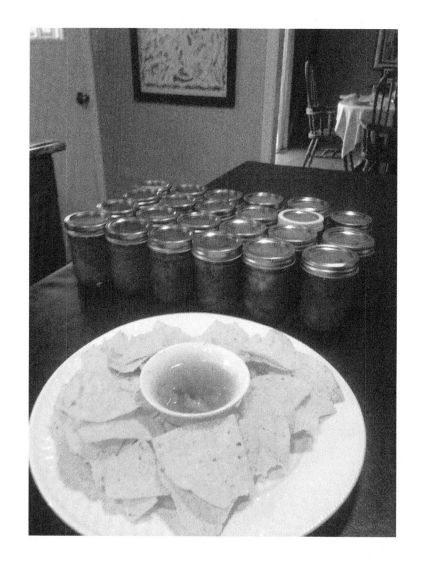

Mango, Pineapple and Habanero Sauce

Grilled pineapple makes this sauce. It adds a unique flavor.

4 cups sugar
1 cup pineapple juice
3 tablespoons lemon juice
1 large pineapple, peeled, sliced and grilled, diced fine
1medium onion, diced fine
1 red pepper, diced fine
1 mango, peeled and diced fine
6 habanero peppers, seeds removed and chopped fine
1 teaspoon xanthan gum
½ cup water

Mix the sugar, vinegar, pineapple juice and lemon juice in a large pot and bring to a boil to dissolve the sugar. Cook for about 2 minutes.

Add the diced pineapple, diced onion, diced peppers and diced mango.

Mix the xanthan gum with the water and stir to soften the xanthan gum then add to the pot with the sugar, peppers etc.

Bring to a boil and then reduce the heat and cook for 1 hour. Stir frequently to avoid scorching.

This can be canned in a hot water bath for 15 minutes.

Balsamic Dressing

This recipe works well with Balsamic vinegars including white and raspberry.

½ cup extra virgin olive oil
½ cup balsamic wine vinegar
2 tablespoons sugar (more if you find it to be too tart, up to ½ cup)
2 teaspoons Dijon mustard
¼ dried oregano
¼ teaspoon thyme
¼ ground white pepper

In a jar with a tight lid (like a canning jar) mix all ingredients and shake well. Store in refrigerator taking out about 1 hour before using to let the olive oil soften to room temperature.

Gorgonzola Dressing

This was a favorite in our restaurant. Play with the seasonings to get it the way you like it, but it was crazy popular! You can substitute blue cheese if you prefer it.

1 cup mayonnaise NOT SALAD DRESSING
½ cup sour cream
½ teaspoon salt
½ teaspoon white pepper
1 teaspoon garlic powder
1 tablespoon onion powder
1 teaspoon Worcestershire sauce (check that it is gluten free)
Dash or 2 of hot pepper sauce
1 cup crumbled gorgonzola cheese

Mix the mayonnaise, sour cream, salt, white pepper, garlic powder, onion powder, Worcestershire sauce and hot pepper sauce well. Fold in the cheese being careful not to over mix. Store in the refrigerator.

Hot Bacon Dressing

Hot Bacon Dressing is generally used on Spinach Salad. It is good on other salads also. Warm it slightly or use cold over your favorite lettuces and fresh vegetables. The bacon is not necessary if you do not prefer pork, just simply omit it from the recipe.

⅔ cup olive oil
¼ cup red wine vinegar
2 tablespoon gluten free soy sauce
2 teaspoons lemon juice
1 teaspoon sugar
1 teaspoon dry mustard
½ teaspoon curry powder
½ teaspoon salt
½ teaspoon white pepper
¼ teaspoon garlic powder
2 tablespoons diced cooked bacon

Combine oil, vinegar, soy sauce, lemon juice, sugar and spices in pan and cook until sugar dissolves and is bubbly. Take of the heat and add bacon. Cool slightly. Serve warm on salad.

This dressing can be stored in an air tight container in the refrigerator for up to 1 week. You can omit the bacon and store up to 1 month adding the bacon to the salad before serving. Heat the dressing slightly before dressing the salad or serve cold if you prefer.

Salsa

½ pound hot peppers (I use a combination of jalapeno, cayenne, cow horn and hot banana peppers).
1 large Spanish onion
4 cloves garlic
3 stalks celery
6 Roma tomatoes, chopped (or green peppers if you like a sweeter salsa)
28 ounce can crushed tomatoes
5.5 ounce can tomato paste
¼ cup water
¼ cup cider vinegar
2.5 teaspoon cumin
1.5 teaspoon salt
2 tablespoons brown sugar (omit if you want a hotter sauce or do not eat sugar)
1 teaspoon dried sweet basil

Chop peppers, celery, onion, tomato and garlic in a small dice. Put all ingredients in a large pot stir. Bring to a boil then reduce to low and cook for 3-4 hours. Stir frequently to prevent scorching. Let stand until internal temperature of 140 and then refrigerate. You can enjoy warm or cold.

This salsa can also be canned in a hot water bath.

Pineapple Salsa

This is fantastic on fish, chicken and pork tenderloin. At our restaurant we served it over pork tenderloin.

The zest of 1 orange
The juice of 1 orange
¼ cup finely diced red onion
2 teaspoons lime juice
¼ teaspoon white pepper
½ teaspoon red pepper sauce
½ cup shredded pineapple, drained well
⅛ teaspoon paprika
⅛ teaspoon salt

Mix all ingredients and use to top cooked pork tenderloin, chicken or a flaky white fish. This salsa can be used warm or cold.

Carne Asada Sauce

This is my favorite marinade! I use this for everything. When in Mexico, I ordered Carne Asada at a restaurant off the tourist path to compare mine with what you can get in Mexico. I was thrilled that this recipe tasted so authentic! You can double or triple the recipe and store it in a canning jar in the refrigerator for future use. When storing it in the refrigerator, remember to take it out about an hour before you need it so the olive oil can soften and then, with the lid on, shake really well as it separates. When the sauce is separated, the olive oil layer should be about the same size as the soy sauce layer. It is perfect as a London broil marinade, use with thinly sliced beef for Carne Asada Tacos or mix into ground beef for nachos or tacos.

⅓ cup white vinegar
½ cup gluten free low sodium soy sauce
2 cloves garlic, chopped
2 tablespoons lime juice
½ cup olive oil
1 teaspoon salt
2 teaspoons black pepper
1 teaspoon garlic powder
½ teaspoon chili powder
1 teaspoon dried oregano
½ teaspoon ground cumin
½ teaspoon paprika

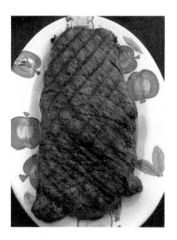

Mix all ingredients and use as a sauce or marinade meat. When using for London Broil, marinate the meat for at least 8 hours before grilling.

London Broil Marinade and Sauce

This was a favorite of my father in law, Hank Babbitt. It is wonderful how great recipes can lead to great memories of those we have lost and miss...

1 cup red wine
2 tablespoons vinegar
2 tablespoons brown sugar
3 tablespoon soy sauce (gluten free)
2 tablespoons olive oil
2 green onions thinly sliced
1 garlic clove, minced
3 pounds top round steak or London Broil steak

Mix all ingredients in a glass or plastic bowl reserving out about ½ cup for basting and add steak.

Marinate for 12-24 hours in refrigerator.

Store the reserve marinade in refrigerator also.

Then grill or broil the steak to desired doneness. Baste with sauce while cooking.

BBQ Sauce

I have used this BBQ sauce for years. It is great on chicken, beef, pork and combined with jams for a different flavor twist. I generally make a large batch and can small jars for use later. This sauce also freezes well if you are not comfortable canning. Just freeze in a small bag with all the air squeezed out.

Check that all ingredients are gluten free!

½ cup firmly packed brown sugar
2 teaspoons salt
2 teaspoons celery seed
½ teaspoon minced garlic
3 cups ketchup
1 cup finely chopped onions
¼ cup lemon juice
¼ cup Worcestershire sauce (check that it is gluten free)
2 teaspoons prepared mustard
1 teaspoon mustard seed

In a large sauce pan, mix all ingredients. Bring to a boil, then reduce heat to a simmer and cook for 20 minutes.

Use immediately on any meat or refrigerate for later use. This sauce is best if made the day before so the flavors can blend.

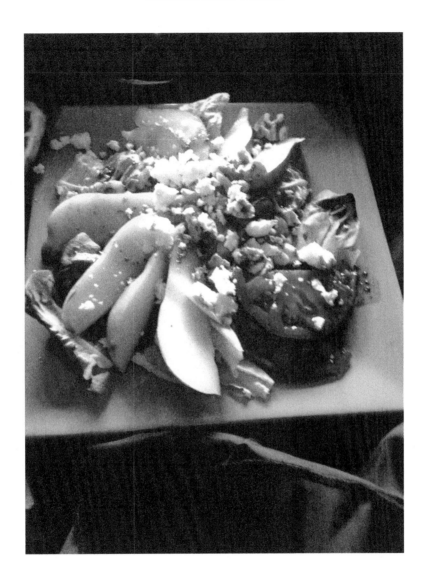

Pear Salad with Walnuts and Feta

This beautiful salad, pictured on previous page, is perfect for dinner parties or just when you want something special for dinner. Feel free to add other fruits and vegetables that you love.

I love this salad with the Raspberry Vinaigrette under the dressings and sauces section page 46. Omit the tomato and it is nightshade free also. I use Bartlett and red pears to add interest and color.

20 (about) walnut halves
Mixed baby greens of your choice
2 Bartlett pears (or other pear variety of your liking)
2 ounces of Feta cheese
1 tomato sliced

Cut the pears into halves or quarters and core the pears. Cut the pears in strips lengthwise. It is beautiful if you keep the halves together and place them over the lettuce and then fan the slices out.

Spread the greens on the bottom of a plate. Top with the pears, walnuts, and tomato and feta cheese.

Top with dressing of your choice, a balsamic tastes great.

Makes 4 salads

Cranberry and Mixed Greens

This is a personal favorite! Change the ingredients up if you have other favorites that you like on salads better. Try this salad with the Raspberry Vinaigrette dressing on page 46.

1 package of mixed greens.
¼ cup red onions diced fine
½ cup green peppers, diced fine
½ cup carrots diced fine
½ cup dried cranberries
¼ cup slivered almonds
1 tomato sliced or cherry tomatoes
4 six ounce chicken breasts, grilled or broiled and sliced
½ cup feta cheese

Divide the mixed greens between 4-6 plates, depending on the size of salad you desire. Top with remaining vegetable ingredients, dividing between the plates. Fan the chicken strips over the salad and top with feta cheese. Drizzle dressing over the salad and serve.

An interesting variation to this salad is instead of using grilled chicken, use the London broil marinated with the Carne Asada Marinade.

Feel free to adjust the amounts of the various foods. I typically use more dried cranberries and almonds on mine...

Spinach Salad

10 ounces of fresh spinach, torn and stems removed
½ pound cooked bacon
2 hard cooked eggs, sliced
½ cup shredded cheese

Place spinach in a large bowl and gently toss with the Hot Bacon Dressing page 47.

Top with the bacon, eggs and shredded cheese and serve.

You can plate the salad separately if you wish. Just toss the spinach and dressing prior to plating in individual servings and then top with cheese, bacon and eggs.

6-8 servings

Wild Rice Salad

1 cup uncooked wild rice
Seasoning salt to taste, optional (check that it is gluten free)
2 cups diced cooked chicken
1 ½ cup green grapes, halved
1 can sliced water chestnuts, drained
¾ cup mayonnaise (you can use light if you prefer, not salad dressing)
1 cup cashews (optional)
1 cup chopped kale or Napa cabbage

Cook rice according to the package directions with seasoned salt (if using). When done, Put in refrigerator to cool.

Place into a large bowl and add remaining ingredients. Mix well and serve chilled.

Greek Salad

This fantastic salad is also great in a gluten free tortilla wrap! Be selective on your Greek dressing, it will matter in the overall flavor. Should you not like Greek dressing, that is okay, just choose one that goes with the flavors in the salad.

4 grilled chicken breasts four to six ounces each
1 cup spinach, stems removed and tear the leaves.
1 bag baby mixed greens or "butter crunch" greens
¼ cup thinly sliced red onion
16 Kalamata olives (approximately 4 for each salad)
1 tomato, sliced
1 cup fresh mushrooms, sliced
6 artichoke hearts chopped (canned, approximately 1 ½ per salad sliced).
½ cup shredded mozzarella cheese
½ cup feta cheese (more or less depending on your taste)

Grill the chicken breasts and slice lengthwise.

Divide mixed greens onto 4 plates and then top with spinach, onions, olives, tomatoes, mushrooms and artichoke hearts.

Slice the chicken breasts and fan on top each salad. Finish with mozzarella and feta cheese and dressing.

Serves 4.

German Potato Salad

½ pound bacon
¾ cup chopped onion
2 tablespoons Kathy's GFFM page 18
¼ teaspoon xanthan gum
⅔ cup cider vinegar;
1 ⅓ cup water
¼ cup sugar
1 teaspoon salt
⅛ teaspoon white pepper
6 cups sliced, peeled, cooked potatoes

Stir the flour and xanthan gum in a small bowl.
In a large skillet, fry the bacon until crisp; remove and set aside.
Drain all but about 3 tablespoons of the bacon drippings and grease.
Cook onions in the bacon grease, drippings until tender.
Stir in the flour and xanthan gum mixture and blend well.
Add the vinegar and water; cook and stir until bubbly and slightly thick.
Cook for 2 minutes stirring constantly.
Add sugar and stir until it dissolves.
Crumble bacon and gently stir in bacon and potatoes.
Heat through, stirring lightly to coat potato slices.
Serve while warm.

Makes 6-8 servings

Broccoli Salad

This was a favorite at our restaurant in Decatur Alabama.

1 bunch (three stalks) of broccoli; cut the flowerets off the stalks and wash
⅓ cup onion
⅓ cup golden raisins (or regular raisins if you prefer)
¼ cup shredded carrots
¼ cup red onion chopped fine
3 tablespoons chopped bacon
1 cup mayonnaise
⅓ cup sugar
2 tablespoons balsamic vinegar
½ teaspoon celery seed

Combine the broccoli flowerets, onion, raisins, carrots and bacon in a large bowl.

In another bowl combine the mayonnaise, sugar, and vinegar and celery seed.

Mix well

Top the broccoli mixture with the dressing and stir well.

Makes 6-8 servings

To add variety, add chicken, grapes, water chestnuts, cashews and kale (or Napa cabbage) to the broccoli salad.

Bean Salad

This is another recipe that I got from my grandmother. We had large family gatherings and being Polish, she made more than enough food for everyone!

Check that all the beans are gluten free.
1 can cut green beans
1 can black beans
1 can cannellini beans
1 can garbanzo beans
1 can navy beans
1 can wax beans
1 large green pepper, chopped
2 celery stalks, chopped
1 jar (2 ounce) pimento, drained
1 bunch green onions, chopped
2 cups vinegar
2 cups sugar
½ cup water
1 teaspoon salt

Drain and rinse all the cans of beans and place in a large bowl.
Add the green pepper, celery, pimento and green onions and set aside.

Mix the vinegar, sugar, water and salt in a sauce pan and bring to a boil. Stir to dissolve the sugar and then pour over the bean mixture. Stir well and refrigerate overnight.

Makes 12 servings so it is perfect for holiday celebrations!

Honey Salad Ambrosia

This was one of my grandmother's favorites.

⅓ cup honey (local is best)
½ cup mayonnaise (light works too)
½ cup walnuts, chopped
3 cored, peeled and chopped granny smith apples
1 small can mandarin oranges
1 cup red (or green) seedless grapes
1 cup mini marshmallows
1 tablespoon lemon juice

Blend the honey and mayonnaise until smooth

Stir the remaining ingredients with the lemon juice and then stir in the mayonnaise mixture.

Refrigerate until ready to serve.

Serves 4-6

Strawberry Pretzel Salad

For those of us in the south Strawberry Pretzel Salad is really popular. Now with the good gluten free pretzels on the market we can now enjoy it too. Those from the North, take a leap of faith, but be careful, it can be addicting. I speak from experience…

Crust:

4 cups gluten free pretzels, crushed fine to 2 cups.
¼ cup sugar
1 stick butter, melted

Filling

1 package of strawberry gelatin (6 ounce size)
2 cups boiling water
1 ½ cup cold water
1 cup chopped fresh strawberries or 1 cup drained, thawed frozen strawberries

Topping:

1 8 ounce tub frozen whipped topping, thawed
4 ounces cream cheese at room temperature
½ cup powdered sugar

Make the gelatin early in the day of the day you will be serving this dish. The gelatin needs to be nearly set when adding the strawberries and then pour on top of the crust. When the gelatin is too thin then the crust will get soggy quickly, and if too set then it will remain chunky and not as attractive.

Boil 2 cups of water and add the gelatin, stirring until dissolved. Add 1 ½ cup cold water and refrigerate for about 1 ½ -2 hours. When just about set, add the strawberries. The frozen strawberries actually work better in this recipe, just strain off all of the juice you can. However, fresh is good too if that is your preference.

Mix the crushed pretzels with the melted butter and sugar. Press into the bottom of a prepared 9x9 or 9x11 inch pan. Bake on 350 for about 10-12 minutes until set. Remove from the oven and cool.

Pour the strawberry gelatin mixture over the cooled crust when the gelatin is just about set. It should not be firm and set up completely, just beginning to set so that when you stir it there is some resistance and setting up. Return to the refrigerator to finish setting up the strawberry layer

Make the topping:

Whip the cream cheese until no lumps remain.

Add the sugar and whip

Add the thawed whipped topping and cover the set strawberry filling.

Keep refrigerated and serve the same day as it is made. The crust will begin to get soggy by the next day.

Sautéed Carmel Apples

I love this recipe!

4 apples.
¼ cup maple syrup
2 teaspoons cinnamon
2 tablespoons coconut oil
½ teaspoon salt

Core and slice apples. Depending on the apple, you can peel the apple or leave the skin on. I make mine with Granny Smith Apples and prefer the skins off.

In a large nonstick skillet mix the syrup, cinnamon, vanilla and coconut oil.

When mixed thoroughly, add the apples. Stir to cover the apples completely with the syrup mixture. Bring the mixture to a boil and then cover and reduce heat.

Simmer on low for 6-10 minutes depending on the apple and the degree of doneness you like.

Remove from heat and add vanilla and salt.

Let the apples stand at room temperature for about 10 minutes or serve hot. The syrup will continue to thicken as it stands.

Serves 4-6 people depending on the size of the apples.

Sautéed Green Beans with Garlic

1 pound fresh green beans, washed
1 tablespoons minced shallots
2 tablespoons olive oil (or coconut oil)
¼ teaspoon salt
¼ teaspoon cracked black pepper
1 minced garlic clove

Wash and trim green beans. Haricot Verts work best in this recipe, if using them snapping is not necessary.

In a Sautee pan, heat oil and add shallots and green beans. Dust with salt and pepper

Cook for about 2 minutes tossing or stirring to prevent burning.

Reduce heat, add garlic and cover the pan for about 2 additional minutes, or longer if you prefer your beans more tender. Remember to remove cover and stir or leave the cover on and shake frequently to prevent the beans from burning.

Sautéed Asparagus and Leeks.

Leeks are among the onion family and are a personal favorite of mine.

Use the above recipe, just make the following substitution:

1 bunch of asparagus, washed and the bottoms snapped off,

1 leek, chop the white only and wash really well.

Follow the above directions for sautéing the asparagus.

Broccoli Casserole

8 cups broccoli florets and peeled, chopped stalks (or combination broccoli and cauliflower)
1 stick butter
½ cup chopped leeks or onions
2 cloves garlic, minced
3 tablespoons Kathy's GFFM page 18
¼ teaspoon xanthan gum
1 ½ cup heavy whipping cream
2 teaspoons Dijon mustard
2 cups chicken or vegetable stock (check gluten free)
1 teaspoon salt and 1 teaspoon pepper
¼ cup parmesan cheese
8 ounces Swiss cheese, shredded
2 cups crushed Chex cereal, rice or corn (optional)

Preheat oven to 400°F

Cook the broccoli (and cauliflower if using) in a steamer or boiling water for about 3 minutes, just until they are beginning to get tender. Drain and pour into a casserole pan.

In a large skillet, melt the butter and add the leeks (or onion) and garlic. Cook for 2 minutes, to sweat. Mix the flour with the cream and add to the onions and garlic and bring to a boil. Add 1 cup of stock. Reserve the additional stock to thin as it cooks so it doesn't get to thick. It should be the consistency of paste. Reduce the heat to medium and cook for 4 minutes to thicken and cook out the starch taste.

Add the mustard, salt, pepper and to the cream mixture and stir well. Add the cheeses and stir until melted in. Pour over the broccoli/ cauliflower. Top with crushed Chex cereal if you are using the cereal for crunch.

Place casserole in the oven and bake until cheese is melted and the sauce is bubbly, about 20 minutes. Serves 6-8 People

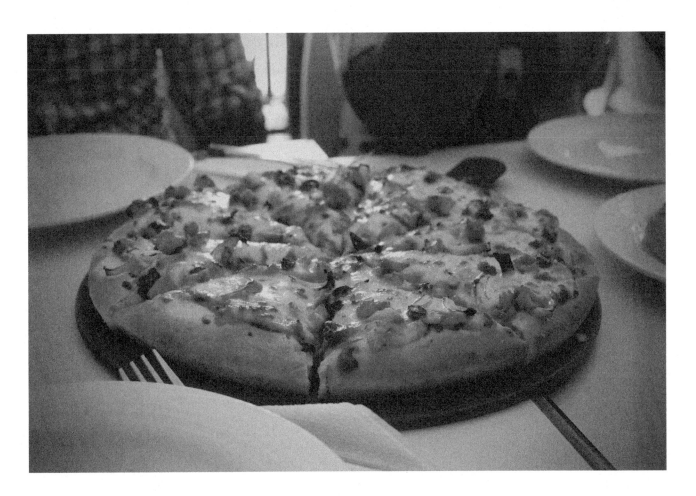

Pizza Crust

This is one of the most requested recipes I get. It is so hard to find a good pizza crust that is gluten free. There are some chain pizza restaurants offering gluten free crusts, but cross contamination is a serious concern if they are also making wheat crusts and using wheat flour to dust work surfaces… Unless it is a gluten free restaurant or bakery, you may be putting yourself at risk to be glutened…You must use a stand mixer for this recipe.

Ingredients:

2 cups Kathy's GFFM page 18
1 teaspoon baking powder
¾ teaspoon salt
1 ½ teaspoon xanthan gum

¾ cup milk (almond milk for dairy free)
¼ cup water
1 ½ teaspoon instant yeast
1 tablespoon honey
2 tablespoons olive oil

1 tablespoon olive oil (in addition to the olive oil listed above)

Place first 4 ingredients in the bowl of a stand mixer and mix until completely blended. Separate out ½ cup of the flour mixture to add to the milk mixture in the next step.

Heat milk and water to 100°F. Add the honey, yeast, 2 tablespoons of olive oil and the ½ cup of the flour mixture. Stir. It is alright if there are large lumps. Set aside for about 15 to 30 minutes until it is bubbly and smells like yeast.

Add the milk mixture to the flour mixture using a stand mixer. Mix until incorporated and then beat on medium speed for 4 minutes. The dough will be thick and really sticky. It will look like thick paste. It will not resemble pizza dough made with wheat flour. Cover and set aside for 30 minutes.

Preheat the oven to 425°F.

Grease a 12 or 14 inch round pizza pan with either gluten free pan spray or vegetable oil. The 12 inch pizza pan will give you a thicker crust.

Drizzle the remaining 1 tablespoons of oil in the center of the pizza pan. Scrape the dough from the bowl onto the oil. The trick to spreading the dough out onto the pan is to drizzle a little olive over the dough and then use plastic wrap to spread it out. Take a piece of plastic wrap and place it over the dough. Using your fingers, move the dough, under the plastic wrap, from the center of the pan to the edges. You may have to move the plastic wrap a couple times, make sure it is not sticking and if it is, add a little more olive oil.

You can also use wet fingers to spread out the dough, but it is really messy (I drizzle a little more olive oil on the dough when it is spread out some). Starting at the center of the dough, push the dough out to the edges of the pan. The dough is still really sticky. You will have to keep wetting your fingers to get it to spread out if you use this method.

Let the dough rest for 15 minutes.

Bake the crust for 10 minutes until set and opaque. Remove from the oven and top with your favorite sauce and toppings.

Return to the oven and finish baking, 10 to 15 minutes depending on your toppings and how thick the toppings are. When the cheese is bubbly and browning it is done.

Salmon Fillets with Mushroom Ragout

6 eight ounce salmon fillets
Fresh lemon juice
2 tablespoons melted butter
Salt and pepper to taste

3 tablespoons butter (in addition to the butter listed above)
3 shallots, minced
2 cups minced fresh mushrooms (use a mixture of your favorites)
½ cup clam juice
¾ cup dry chardonnay
¼ cup whipping cream
½ teaspoon tarragon

Preheat oven to 450°F
Place salmon, skin side down, on a nonstick baking sheet.
Mix the lemon juice and melted butter. Brush the salmon with the butter, lemon juice and lightly dust with salt and pepper. Bake until done, about 12-15 minutes. Be careful to not overcook.

While cooking the salmon, prepare the mushroom ragout:

Melt the butter in a heavy large skillet over medium heat and add the shallots. Cook for about 2 minutes. Turn the heat to medium high and add in the mushrooms. Sauté until beginning to brown, about 7-8 minutes stirring constantly to prevent burning. Do not heat to high, you do not want to burn the butter or the shallots.

Add the clam juice and wine. Boil until you reduce the liquid by about half. Keep warm while the salmon is finishing.

When the salmon is done, plate the salmon, and add the cream to the mushroom mixture, stirring to make it creamy. Season ragout with salt and pepper and top the salmon with the sauce and serve.

6 servings.

Herb Crusted Cod

4 cod fillets (about 16 ounces of fish. This can be one fillet or 4 smaller fillets)
1 cup of gluten free bread crumbs
2 cloves of garlic, crushed
The zest of 1 lemon
1 tablespoon fresh chives
1 tablespoon chopped fresh parsley
1 tablespoon chopped fresh basil
Dash of coarse salt
Dash of pepper
2 tablespoons extra virgin olive oil

Preheat the oven to 400°F

Line a cookie sheet with parchment or lightly grease the pan to prevent sticking.

Place the bread crumbs in a shallow dish.

Chop the parsley, garlic, lemon zest, chives, and basil and add the bread crumbs. Stir to combine.

Brush the top of the cod with olive oil and then dip into the bread crumbs.

Place in prepared pan, crust side up and bake until firm, about 12-15 minutes.

Serves 4

Gorgonzola Shrimp and Spinach

28 Shrimp (7 per person, this is just a suggestion and depends on the size of the shrimp)
¼ cup butter (clarified or Gee works best)
1 can artichoke hearts, drained and chopped
1 cup fresh spinach, packed firmly, chopped
1 green or red pepper sliced thinly
1 medium onion, sliced thinly
2 cups seafood stock or vegetable stock (check that it is gluten free)
2 cups whipping cream
¼ cup Kathy's GFFM page 18
½ cup gorgonzola cheese
Adzuki bean pasta, cooked by package instructions and cooled.

Cook pasta and set aside.

Melt butter in a very large sauté pan or pot and add shrimp. Be very careful not to brown the butter if not using clarified butter or Gee (butter cooked at too high a temperature will burn easily). Cook them all at the same time if possible, otherwise keep cooked shrimp warm, not hot, while cooking the remaining shrimp. Keep all shrimp warm when finished, not hot, while making the sauce.

Cook the onions, peppers and spinach in the same pan with the same butter as the shrimp. Again, be careful not to scorch the butter if not using clarified or Gee. When the onions and peppers are tender, add the artichoke hearts and stock.

Whisk the whipping cream and the flour in a bowl and add to the vegetables cooking in the skillet. Bring to a boil, turn the heat down and simmer for 4 minutes to thicken and cook out the starch taste.

When the sauce is done toss in the shrimp and the pasta to heat through. Top with Gorgonzola cheese.

Serves 4-6 depending on how many shrimp you cook.

Tuna and Salsa Verde

This is another recipe from our restaurant. Customers loved it!

4 tuna steaks (or 2 larger steaks, enough for 4 people)
¼ cup olive oil
2 teaspoons lemon juice
Salt and pepper
2 teaspoons anchovy paste
1 cup flat leaf parsley leaves
½ ounce fresh mint
1 tablespoons chopped capers
1 teaspoon Dijon mustard
1 tablespoon white wine
½ cup olive oil

Combine olive oil and lemon juice in a plastic bag and place steaks in the bag to marinate for about 15 minutes. Make the salsa while the tuna marinades.

In a food processor combine anchovy paste, flat leaf parsley, and mint, capers, mustard and white wine. Turn the processor on and pulse until all ingredients are mixed and chopped fine. With the processor running, pour the olive oil into the processor in a slow thin stream. Continue to process until smooth.

Cook tuna steaks. Heat the grill or skillet and when hot, add the tuna. Cook for about 2 minutes and then turn and cook the other side about 2 minutes.

Move the tuna away from the hottest part of the grill, or turn the heat of the skillet down and finish cooking about 8 minutes. How long you cook the tuna will depend on the type of tuna and your preference for doneness. Ahi tuna cooked rare is done after shortly after searing for example. When tuna is done top with the salsa Verde and serve.

Makes 4 servings

Herb Crusted Pork Chops

Tender and juicy. Serve with sautéed apples or Brussel sprouts for a nutritious dinner.

2-4 pork chops, bone in or boneless as you prefer. Do not trim fat.
3 tablespoons Dijon style mustard
2 tablespoon chopped fresh thyme
2 teaspoons chopped fresh oregano
2 teaspoons dried parsley
½ teaspoon white pepper
½ teaspoon salt
1 tablespoon light refined olive oil or coconut oil

Preheat oven to 375°F.

Rinse the pork chops and then pat dry with paper towels.

Mix the thyme, oregano, parsley, pepper and salt together on a plate.

Spread the mustard on the pork chops and then press the pork chops into the herb mixture.

Heat the oil in an oven proof skillet. When the oil is hot, add the chops and sear on each side for 2 minutes per side.

Transfer the pan to the oven to finish cooking. The cook time will depend on the thickness of the pork chop. It should take about 8 minutes for a thin chop (1/4 inch) up to 20 minutes for a 1 inch chop. Check frequently though, as pork will over cook very easily!

Cook until the internal temperature is 135-140°F. **<u>Use a thermometer</u>**. They will continue to cook after removing from the oven. You can cook to 145°F if you are concerned about the temperature, but it will result in a dryer chop.

Let stand for 10 minutes. DO NOT CUT IT STRAIGHT FROM THE OVEN. Cutting it too soon will result in all of the juices draining from the chop and it will be dry.

Fennel and White beans

2 tablespoons light refined olive oil
4 cups kale washed and chopped
1 large fennel bulb washed and chopped
1 pound of presoaked and precooked navy beans or other white beans*
1-2 cups of chicken stock
Parmesan cheese (optional)
Jalapeno pepper chopped and seeds removed
Salt and pepper to taste

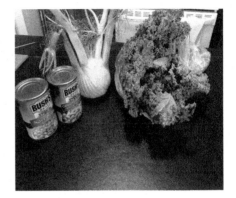

Drizzle the olive oil in a hot skillet and add the chopped kale and fennel.

Cook until the kale is wilted and fennel is tender.

Add the beans, jalapeno pepper and chicken stock.

Add salt and pepper to taste.

Turn the heat to low and simmer for 15-20 minutes, stirring occasionally, until beans are cooked through and the chicken stock has reduced down. It will thicken as it cooks.

Serve when warm and top with parmesan cheese or other white cheese you desire.

Make 4 -6 servings.

* 1 pound of raw beans cooks to 2 pounds of beans. You can also use 2 cans of beans. Check that they are gluten free.

Pinto Beans with Smoked Sausage

2 cans canned pinto beans; check that they are gluten free
2 small onions chopped
6 ounces beef sausage, cut into 1 inch chunks (check that it is gluten free)
2 cups chopped kale (optional)
½ teaspoon salt
½ teaspoon white pepper
1 chopped jalapeno pepper
½ teaspoon chopped garlic
¼ teaspoon cayenne pepper
1 cup unsalted chicken stock (check that it is gluten free)
2 tablespoons light refined olive oil

Sauté kale in olive oil for about 5 minutes and then add onions and sausage. Cook until sausage is browned and the onion is tender and then add jalapeno pepper. Cook for another 5 minutes and add garlic, seasoning and chicken stock. Add beans and cook for another 10 minutes until some of the stock has evaporated and has thickened. Serve on rice or alone with bread.

Makes 4-6 servings

Raspberry BBQ Chicken Wings

2 pounds Chicken wings, separated
½ BBQ sauce (recipe from Sauces & Dressing chapter)
½ cup Raspberry Jam

Preheat oven to 400°F if baking wings.

Bake or fry wings (you can also buy the wings, cooked from most large supermarkets). Make sure they are "naked" wings. This just means that they are not breaded. Also, check with the deli staff or manager that the chicken is not cooked with foods that are breaded in the same oil.

Separate drumettes and wing tips.

Set a wire rack inside of a cookie sheet and spread them out in a single layer. Bake wings until cooked and the skin is crispy, about 45-50 minutes.

Mix the BBQ sauce and raspberry jam in a small sauce pan and heat to a boil. Turn off the heat and let set.

When the chicken is done, place the chicken wings in a shallow baking pan. Top with sauce and bake for 10-15 minutes to set the sauce.

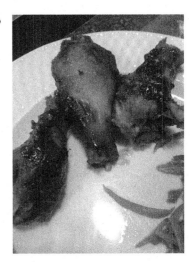

Serve while still hot, or chill and eat cold.

Chicken and Capers

We served this in our Restaurant and it was consistently a favorite. This is very easy and quick to make at home. Serve with sautéed asparagus or sautéed green beans for a perfect dinner. Serve over gluten free pasta or rice.

4-6 boneless and skinless chicken breasts (approximately 6 ounce, pound so they are about the same thickness)
¼ cup Kathy's GFFM page 18
2 tablespoons light refined olive oil
1 tablespoon butter
1 tablespoon capers, chopped
1 tablespoon green onions, chopped
¼ teaspoon tarragon
½ cup dry chardonnay
1 cup heavy cream
2 tablespoons Kathy's GFFM (this is in addition to the amount above.)
Salt and pepper to taste
Parmesan cheese, optional
Additional chopped green onions for garnish, optional

Preheat oven to 400°F.

Place the GF flour in a flat pan or plate and dredge the chicken breasts in the flour. This step is optional, but it does help the sauce to stick to the chicken.

Place olive oil in a hot skillet and add the chicken. Cook for 2 minutes on each side and place the chicken in the preheated oven to finish cooking, about 7-10 minutes.

Add the butter to a small sauce pan and melt. Add the chopped capers, chopped green onions and tarragon. Lightly sauté the capers, green onions and tarragon in the butter. Be careful not to scorch the butter or use clarified butter. The butter should not turn brown.

Sauté for about 2 minutes and then add white wine. Simmer to reduce the wine by half.

Mix the heavy cream and flour in a bowl with a wire whisk and add to the wine mixture.

Cook, stirring constantly, for about 4 minutes to cook out the starch flavor. Season with salt and pepper to taste.

Pour over the chicken when it has finished cooking.

Serve Hot

4-6 servings

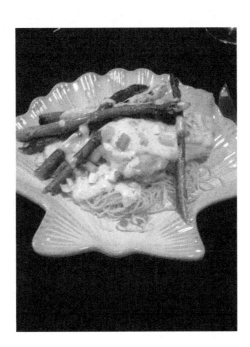

Asian Chicken

Using fresh ingredients like fresh jalapeno peppers, fresh carrots and fresh ginger will make a big difference in this recipe. Always use fresh ginger when you can.

Sauce

1 jalapeno pepper, seeds removed and chopped
1 tablespoon garlic
3 tablespoons brown sugar
½ cup water
2 tablespoons lime juice

Chicken:

1 tablespoon light refined olive oil
1 tablespoon sesame oil
12 ounces boneless skinless chicken breasts cubed
½ cup diced carrots
1 tablespoon minced fresh ginger
1 tablespoon low sodium soy sauce (check that it is gluten free)
1 can water chestnuts, drained
1 cup chicken broth
1 tablespoon corn starch (check that it is gluten free)
1 package gluten free Asian noodles, cooked and cooled

Prepare the sauce by mixing all ingredients and bring to a boil. Turn off the heat and set aside.

Heat a large sauté pan and add olive oil and sesame oil. Add the chicken and cook at medium heat until chicken is turning white, add carrots. Continue cooking until chicken is browned and carrots are starting to get tender.

Mix the chicken broth and cornstarch and whisk until smooth.

Add soy sauce, ginger, water chestnuts, chicken broth (with the cornstarch) and noodles to the chicken mixture.

Cook until the sauce is thickened. Add water or more chicken stock if it is too thick for your tastes.

To serve; place the chicken mixture in a bowl and top with the sauce.

Serve while hot. You can add other vegetables if you wish. Broccoli, snow peas and peppers are great also.

4-6 servings

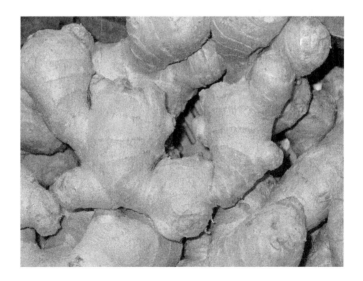

Honey Mustard Chicken

4 six ounce boneless, skinless chicken breasts. Pound with a mallet to approximately the same thickness
½ teaspoon cracked black pepper
¼ teaspoon salt
2 teaspoons light refined olive oil
¼ cup raw honey
¼ cup low sodium gluten free chicken broth
¼ teaspoon dried thyme
1 tablespoon cider vinegar
1 tablespoon Dijon style mustard (stone ground)

Preheat oven to 400°F

Heat a skillet over high heat. Add olive oil to hot pan and swirl to coat

Add chicken, dust with salt and pepper. Sauté chicken about 2 minutes per side and then place on a shallow pan and place in the oven to finish cooking; about 10 minutes.

In a small skillet, combine the honey, thyme, and chicken broth. Bring to a boil and reduce by half while the chicken is cooking. When broth mixture has reduced by about ½, add the vinegar and mustard. Continue to cook stirring occasionally so it does not burn.

After the chicken has cooked about 8 minutes, baste the chicken with the honey mustard and let it finish cooking.

Baste one last time when the chicken has finished and serve hot.

Makes 4 servings.

Spicy Turkey Noodle Soup

Check that all ingredients are gluten free.

1 tablespoon sesame oil
1 pound lean ground turkey breast
2 cloves garlic, finely chopped
1 teaspoon grated fresh gingerroot
2 32 oz. cartons gluten free chicken broth
3 tablespoons gluten free reduced sodium soy sauce
1 tablespoon lime juice
2 teaspoons hot pepper sauce like Sriracha sauce
1 ½ teaspoons red curry paste
1 cup snow peas
½ cup carrots, chopped
1 red bell pepper cut into strips
1 green bell pepper cut into strips
Any other vegetables that you wish
3 ounces uncooked rice noodles

Heat oil in saucepan and cook (stirring frequently) the turkey, garlic and gingerroot until turkey is no longer pink.

Add broth, soy sauce, lime juice, Sriracha and red curry paste and simmer for 5 minutes. Sir in vegetables and uncooked noodles and cook until about 8-10 more minutes until vegetables are tender.

Adjust seasonings to taste and serve hot.

Makes 6-8 servings

Crespella Alla Bolognese

Bolognese Filling

2 tablespoon butter
1 tablespoon olive oil
1 onion, chopped
16 ounces ground beef
1 small green pepper chopped
8 ounce can diced tomatoes
1 tablespoon tomato paste
8 ounces beef stock (check that it is gluten free)
1 cup water
2 teaspoons dried basil
1 teaspoon dried oregano
Salt and pepper to taste

Sauce

1 tablespoon butter
1 onion chopped
1 16 ounce can diced tomatoes
Salt and pepper to taste
1 tablespoon basil leaves
You can omit this step and use your favorite GF Tomato Pasta Sauce.

Crepes

¾ cup Kathy's GFFM page 18
1 teaspoon xanthan gum
½ teaspoon baking soda
2 large egg
1 ½ cup milk
1 teaspoon vanilla
2 tablespoons (approximately) oil, coconut, light refined olive oil or vegetable.

Directions

Preheat oven to 400°F

To make the Bolognese Filling, brown the beef with onions in a skillet over medium heat. After meat browned with onions, mix in all remaining filling ingredients and simmer 45 minutes.

To make the Crepes; while the filling is simmering, mix the dry ingredients in a bowl and whisk to blend. Then mix the wet ingredients together. Add the wet ingredients to the dry ingredients. Stir to incorporate all ingredients and let stand for 5 minutes before cooking.

Heat about 2 tablespoons of oil in a small nonstick skillet. After the oil is melted, swirl to coat the pan and then pour out the excess into a heat proof bowl or coffee mug. Use this oil for the other crapes you will make in the pan. Using a ¼ cup measuring cup, drop the batter in the hot nonstick skillet. The crapes should be very thin. After adding the batter to the pan, pick up the pan and swirl it to spread the batter out as thin as possible. Let brown slightly then flip the crape and cook until that side is browned also. Remove from heat and then continue with the next crape. Makes 8 crapes.

Make sauce:

Mix all the sauce ingredients together and bring to a boil. Reduce the heat to low and simmer until the onions are tender, about 10 minutes.

Assemble crapes by putting a small amount of the meat filling in the center of the crape and rolling it up (like an enchilada). Place them in a baking pan, seam side down, that has been either greased or sprayed with pan spray so they do not sick to the pan. Pour ½ the sauce over the top of the crapes. Bake in the oven for about 8 minutes at 400°F and top with remaining sauce.

4-6 servings

Gluten Free Lasagna

Sauce:

1 pound ground beef, browned and broken into small pieces
3 15.5 ounce cans tomato sauce
2 tablespoons Italian seasoning
1 teaspoon oregano
2 tablespoons basil
2 teaspoons garlic (to taste or omit if you do not prefer garlic)
1 teaspoon salt
1 teaspoon pepper

Filling:

1 15 ounce container Ricotta cheese
1 egg
1 pound of mozzarella cheese

Noodles

1 pound (1 box) of gluten free lasagna noodles, do not precook.
1 13X9 cake pan (this can be a foil pan, glass or metal)
Foil
Plastic wrap

Cook ground beef breaking it apart as it cooks into small pieces.

When the meat is browned, add all of the sauce ingredients and continue to cook for about 30 minutes. Stir occasionally to prevent scorching.

Mix the Ricotta cheese and the egg in a large bowl.

Layer the lasagna:

1. Ladle some sauce into the bottom of the pan

2. Add 1 layer of noodles

3. Top with ricotta cheese mixture

4. Top with mozzarella cheese

5. Top with more sauce

6. Top with 1 layer of noodles

7. Top with sauce

8. Top with mozzarella cheese

9. Wrap the pan with the plastic wrap followed by the foil. Seal tightly.

Cook at 350°F for 1 hour, carefully remove the foil and then the plastic wrap. Pierce the top of the plastic wrap before removing to let steam escape and avoid a steam burn. This can be done with a long handle knife, long handle fork or tongs.

Return to the oven for another 10-15 minutes to allow the cheese to brown.

Serve hot.

Serves 6-8 depending on the size of the portion.

Chipotle Meatloaf or Meatballs

2 eggs
2 cloves garlic minced
1 chipotle chili in adobe sauce, diced
2 tablespoon adobo sauce from chipotle peppers
1 teaspoon salt
1 teaspoon coarse ground black pepper
½ teaspoon celery seed
½ teaspoon ground cumin
1 tablespoon Worcestershire sauce (check that it is gluten free)
1 tablespoon gluten low sodium free soy sauce
1 onion chopped fine
½ cup gluten free oatmeal
2 pounds lean ground beef
2 tablespoons barbeque sauce (either the one in this book or your own personal favorite)

Preheat oven to 350°F

Beat the eggs in a large mixing bowl until smooth then whisk in the garlic, chilies, sauce, salt, pepper, celery seed, and cumin and Worcestershire sauce.

Add in the remainder of the ingredients and mix with clean hands until well blended. Place meatloaf in either a 8x8 baking pan or a large bread pan and pat down in the pan with your hands or form into meatballs and place on a cookie sheet to bake.

Brush top with additional barbeque sauce if desired

Bake Meatloaf in preheated oven until no longer pink in the center about 1 hour in a 350 degree oven.

Meat balls take considerably less time and cook time varies based on their size.

Instant read thermometer needs to read at 160°F when inserted into the center of the meatloaf.

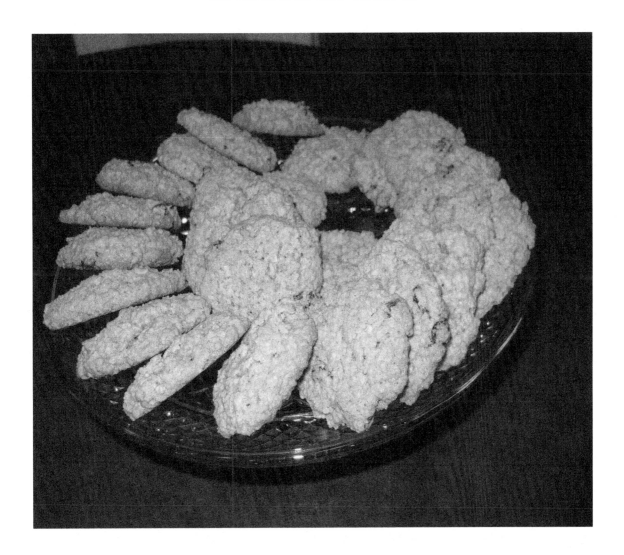

Chocolate Pecan Bars

These are amazingly easy to make and are great to take to a luncheon to share with friends!

Crust

2 cup Kathy's GFFM page 18
1 cup packed brown sugar
1 teaspoon xanthan gum
½ cup salted butter softened

Carmel Filling

½ cup brown sugar (in addition to the amount listed above)
⅔ cup salted butter, (in addition to the amount listed above)
½ cup semi-sweet chocolate chips (1 cup total, divided)

Topping

1 cup pecans (optional)
½ cup semi-sweet chocolate chips
1 teaspoon salt (optional)

Crust: Heat oven to 350°F. Combine flour, xanthan gum, brown sugar, and softened butter in bowl and beat at medium speed until mixture is crumbly. Press into the bottom of a greased 13x9 inch pan.

Filling: Combine ⅔ cup butter and ½ cup brown sugar in a saucepan and cook over medium heat. Stir constantly until the entire surface begins boiling. Continue cooking stirring constantly 1 minute. Pour over the crust mix and carefully spread it evenly over the entire crust avoiding the edges. Pour ½ of the chocolate chips over the caramel and bake.

Bake for 18-20 minutes or until entire caramel layer is bubbly. Do not overbake.

Topping: Remove from the oven and sprinkle with chips, pecans and salt (optional). Allow them to melt and then swirl melted chips over bars.
Cool and then cut into bars. Store at room temperature in a loosely covered container.

No Bake Cookie Recipe

This was a recipe of my grandmother's. Make these when you have someone to share them with. They are amazingly good!

5 cups rice Chex© cereal
1 cup salted peanuts
1 cup sugar
1 cup corn syrup
1 cup peanut butter

Grease a 9x13 inch cake pan.

Pour the cereal and peanuts in the pan.

Place sugar and syrup in a heavy sauce pan and bring to a rolling boil.

Remove from heat as soon as mixture boils.

Add peanut butter and mix well.

Pour over cereal and peanuts and cool.

Cut into squares and Store in a covered container.

Peanut Butter Bars

These are very simple to make and if you watch your ingredient labels, are gluten free!

2 cups peanut butter
1/2 cup melted butter (can use margarine if you prefer)
1 pound (box) powdered sugar
1 teaspoon vanilla

Melt butter, add peanut butter, powdered sugar and vanilla. It will be really hard to mix as it is very dry. Use a stand mixer or mix with clean hands. I use a stand up Kitchen Aid with the paddle or dough hook.

When mixed thoroughly, place in large cookie sheet and cover with wax paper and roll the mixture out with a rolling pin till packed down and the thickness you prefer. Covering the peanut butter mixture with wax paper (or plastic wrap if you prefer) makes rolling easier and prevents the mix from sticking to the rolling pin.

Chocolate topping

2 cups semi-sweet chocolate chips
2 tablespoons butter

Melt in a double boiler or in microwave. When using microwave, melt carefully using short time cycles and stirring often.

Spread over top of peanut butter mixture and let set at room temperature for 1 hour.

Cut into squares and store at room temperature or in refrigerator for longer time periods. They also freeze well.

Peanut Butter Balls

12 ounces chocolate chips
2 ½ cups graham cracker crumbs (gluten free)*
1 cup melted margarine
1 pound powdered sugar
1 cup nuts or rice crispy cereal
1 cup peanut butter

Mix graham cracker crumbs, powdered sugar and nuts or cereal together.

Add peanut butter and melted margarine

Blend well

Using a tablespoon measuring spoon form into balls

Place in the freezer and chill for one hour

Melt the chocolate chips in a double boiler and dip the chilled balls into the melted chocolate

Place on wax paper to set

Makes around 100 balls

The Peanut Butter Balls can be stored for several days in a sealed container in a cool location.

* You might have to purchase gluten free graham crackers and crush them to make crumbs.

Short Bread Cookies

This is a perfect example of why I am writing this cookbook. This recipe was one of my grandmothers. It was a polish donut recipe. It is very old and some would have simply traded the wheat flour for a gluten free flour and think that would be enough. I made the "donuts", doing exactly that. I substituted my gluten free flour blend along with some xanthan gum and it was terrible. The donuts would not rise. No amount of begging would get it done. The original recipe had yeast in it. I baked them anyway and amazingly, they were the best sugar cookies that I have ever had! Perfect for frosting during the holidays!

3 ½ cups Kathy's GFFM page 18
2 teaspoons xanthan gum
1 teaspoon baking powder
⅓ cup butter at room temperature
⅔ cup sugar
1 egg
3 egg yolks
1 teaspoon vanilla
¾ teaspoon salt
1 teaspoon orange and lemon peel (optional)

Mix the gluten free flour, xanthan gum and salt in a bowl with a wire whisk to blend completely.

In the bowl of a stand mixer, cream butter and sugar until fluffy, beat in the whole egg then yolks, adding one at a time

Add vanilla and fruit peel,

Beat until well mixed

Stir in the flour gradually adding enough to make stiff dough

Turn dough onto a flour surface, cover and let stand 20 minutes.

Turn onto lightly floured surface and pat or roll to ¼ inch thickness

Cut out with a cookie cutter

Bake in 350°F for 12-15 minutes until lightly browned.

Let rest on cookie sheet for 10 minutes then transfer to a wire rack to cool. Decorate as you wish.

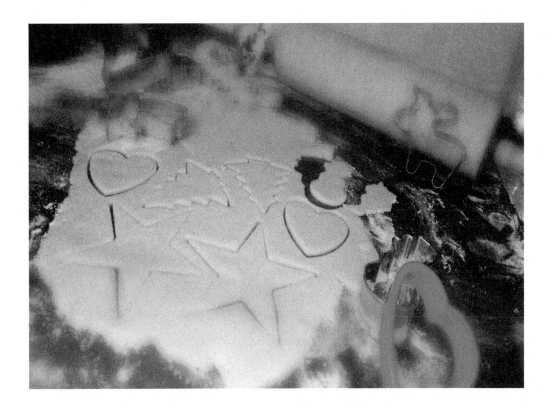

Oatmeal Raisin Cookies

3 cups gluten free old fashioned rolled oats*
½ cup warm water
¾ cup plus 2 tablespoons almond flour
⅔ cup Kathy's GFFM page 18
½ teaspoon salt
½ cup baking powder
½ teaspoon xanthan gum
½ teaspoon nutmeg
½ teaspoon cinnamon
1 cup packed brown sugar
½ cup granulated sugar
8 tablespoons butter
1 large egg
1 egg yolk
2 tablespoons vegetable oil
1 tablespoon vanilla extract
1 cup raisins

Mix oats and water and let stand to soften*

Preheat oven to 325

Whisk flours, salt, baking powder, xanthan gum, spices in a bowl to mix

In a stand mixer mix sugars and butter until light and fluffy, add egg and yolk and mix until well combined and add vanilla.

Stir in flour mixture and mix until smooth.

Mix in oats that have been soaking in water.

Remove from the mixer and fold in the raisins.

Cover the bowl and let stand for 30 minutes.

Line 2 baking sheets with parchment paper.

Roll dough into a ball using a tablespoon and place on the parchment about 2 inches apart, press them flat. These cookies will not spread out so flattening them slightly with the bottom of a glass or metal pancake turner is important.

Cook at 325 degrees in the center of the oven for approximately 22-25 minutes until the edges are beginning to brown and the centers are soft. Turn the cookie sheets while baking to evenly brown.

Cool on the cookies sheet at least 5 minutes before transferring to a wire rack to cool.

*You do not have to soften the oats in water if they are quick cooking oats. Use the same amount of oats, just omit the water.

Chocolate Chip Cookies

1 ½ cup Kathy's GFFM page 18
½ teaspoon baking soda
½ teaspoon salt
¾ teaspoon xanthan gum

8 tablespoons salted butter melted (2 sticks butter)*
¾ cup light brown sugar
2 ⅓ cup white sugar (organic or coconut sugar)

1 large egg
2 tablespoons milk (or Almond Milk if you are dairy free)
1 tablespoon vanilla extract

8 ounces chocolate chips

Preheat oven to 350°

Whisk flour blend, baking soda, salt, xanthan gum together in medium bowl and set aside.

Mix melted butter, brown sugar and sugar in a large bowl until well combined and smooth.

Mix in egg, milk and vanilla and continue to mix until smooth.

Stir in the flour mixture with a rubber spatula until well blended. It should be a soft homogeneous dough.

Fold in the chocolate chips and cover the bowl with plastic wrap and let sit for 30 minutes. The dough will be sticky and soft.

Line 2 baking sheets with parchment paper. Measure out 2 tablespoons of dough and roll into balls.

Space the cookies about 2 inches apart on the prepared sheets.

Bake cookies, 1 sheet at a time in the center of the oven until edges are set and beginning to brown but the centers are still soft, about 11-15 minutes.

Cool on the cookie sheet for 5 minutes before transferring to wire rack to cool. Store in an air tight container for up to 2 days but are best eaten the day cooked. You can also freeze for future enjoyment.

*Use a Gluten Free Dairy Free butter substitute if you are dairy free.

Raspberry Bars

These bars are as good as or better than the gluten filled variety. They are actually Gluten Free and can be Casein free!

¼ cup steel cut GF oats
2 tablespoons milk (or light Almond Milk)
¾ cup quick cooking GF Oatmeal
1 cup Kathy's GFFM page 18
½ teaspoon ground cinnamon
½ teaspoon baking soda
¼ teaspoon salt
½ teaspoon xanthan gum
½ cup butter or margarine (or gluten free dairy free butter substitute)
½ cup packed brown sugar
2 large eggs
1 teaspoon pure vanilla extract (check for gluten free)
¾ cup raspberry preserves

Preheat oven to 350 degrees

Prepare a 13"x9" cake pan with a pan spray (gluten free) or coconut oil.

Measure the steel cut oats into a small bowl and add the 2 tablespoons almond milk, stir and set aside.

Measure the quick cooking gluten free oats, gluten free AP flour, cinnamon, salt and xanthan gum into a medium bowl and whisk to blend. Set aside.

With an electric mixer, beat the margarine (or butter) and the brown sugar until light and fluffy. Add the eggs, one at a time, beating well after each addition. Add the Vanilla.

Gradually add flour mixture and continue mixing. Let stand for 10 minutes.

Remove 1/3 of the batter for topping and spread the remaining in the bottom of the prepared cake pan.

Top with the raspberry preserves, spreading evenly over the batter.

Top with the remaining batter.

Bake for 25-30 minutes until tester comes out clean. Serve warm or cooled and top with glaze if you wish.

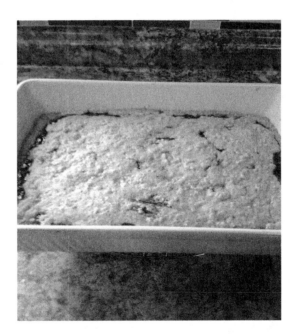

Oatmeal Chocolate Chip Cookies

Your guests will not be able to tell that they are gluten free!

1 ¾ cup gluten free quick cooking oats
1 tablespoon almond flour
1 ¾ cup Kathy's GFFM page 18
1 teaspoon baking soda
1 teaspoon xanthan gum
½ teaspoon salt
½ cup butter (or gluten free margarine or coconut oil)
1 cup dark brown sugar
½ cup granulated white sugar (organic sugar or coconut sugar)
2 large eggs
1 teaspoon gluten free vanilla
2 tablespoons milk (or Almond Milk)
10 ounce gluten free chips about 2 cups (you can use gluten free/dairy free Chocolate chips)

Preheat oven to 375 degree and line cookie sheets with parchment paper.

Mix the oats, almond flour, Kathy's GFFM, baking soda, xanthan gum and salt in bowl with a wire whisk and set aside.

Using an electric mixer, cream together butter and sugars in a large bowl until well blended.

Beat in eggs one at a time. Beat in the vanilla and milk.

Gradually add the dry ingredients beating until well combined. Stir in the chocolate chips.

Using a tablespoon, form each cookie into a ball and place on a prepared cookie sheet. Gently press down on the cookies with the bottom of a glass or a fork (these cookies do not spread out).

Bake cookies in preheated oven about 11 minutes until the edges turn brown .Remove from oven and cool 5 minutes on cookie sheet and then transfer to wire rack to cool completely.

All Gluten Free flours are not created equal. Please use the flour specified when possible. Different blends use different flours. For example, the Falafel bread calls for Bobs Red Mill All Purpose Baking Flour. That is because the fist ingredient is Garbanzo Bean Flour. Using it to make a cake, would make a "bean cake" and that may not be what you had in mind…

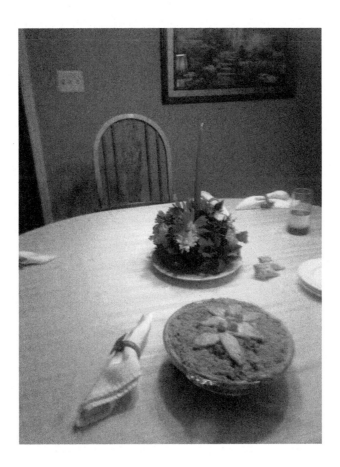

Pina Colada Cheesecake

This is a very flavorful cheesecake that is perfect for special occasions and dinner parties. Remember to mix the cream cheese until there are no lumps remaining! Scrape the bowl and beaters carefully so that you get all the cream cheese whipped. Also the cream cheese needs to be at room temperature. After all the lumps are whipped out, beat in the sugar. Beat the sugar in for several minutes incorporating air into the cheesecake.

1 gluten free graham cracker crust see page 121.
16 ounces cream cheese
1 cup sugar
½ can shredded pineapple drained well
¼ cup coconut
2 eggs
1 tablespoons rum or 1 teaspoon rum extract

Make the crust according to the instructions on page 121.
Preheat oven to 300°F
Whip the cream cheese until no lumps remain.
Add the sugar and beat in completely.
Add the shredded pineapple and coconut and mix well.
Add eggs one at a time and beat well after each egg to make sure it is incorporated completely.
Add flavoring, mixing in completely and pour into a prepared pan and bake at 300 degrees for 1 hour for 8" Pan (50 minutes for 10" spring form pan) before opening the door of the oven.

At 1 hour baking time check the cheese cake for doneness and when the outer 2 inches are done and the center appears set, (it may sill jiggle slightly). Remove from the oven and run a knife around the outside of the pan.

Place the cake in a warm area to cool. Cool in pan completely.

Cut the cheesecake with a wet, sharp knife for best results and serve with whipped cream.

Crème Brule Cheesecake

The secret to a great cheese cake is beating the cream cheese until no lumps remain. Once you add the remaining ingredients the lumps you have will always be there. Also, do not open the oven to check the cheesecake before 50-60 minutes unless you smell it burning. Slight changes in temperature will cause the cheesecake to crack.

1 gluten free graham cracker crust see page 121

Filling:

16 ounces cream cheese at room temperature
½ cup white sugar
2 egg yolks
1 egg
¼ cup whipped cream
½ teaspoon vanilla (gluten free)

Preheat oven to 300°F. Line a spring form pan bottom with parchment cut into a circle and either grease the pan bottom and sides or use GF spray release on the inside the pan.

Make the crust according to instructions on page 121.

Whip the cream cheese until no lumps remain.

Add the sugar and beat in completely.

Add the egg yolks one at a time. Beating well after each addition.

Add whole egg. Beat until completely combined

Beat in whipped cream, mix until completely combined

Add vanilla and mix in completely.

Pour into a prepared pan and bake at 300 degrees for 1 hour for an 8" spring form pan, (50 minutes for 10" spring form pan) before opening the door of the oven.

At 1 hour baking time check the cheese cake for doneness and when the outer 2 inches are done and the center appears set (it may sill jiggle slightly). Remove from the oven and run a knife around the outside of the pan.

Place the cake in a warm area to cool. You can also turn off the oven and open the door leaving the cheesecake in the oven for another 20 minutes to begin cooling. Then remove from the oven and place in a draft free area to cool. When the cheesecake reaches 125 degrees, refrigerate to finish cooling. Cool in pan completely.

Before serving, sprinkle with white sugar and then with a lighter stick or kitchen blow torch heat the sugar until it browns. Cut and serve.

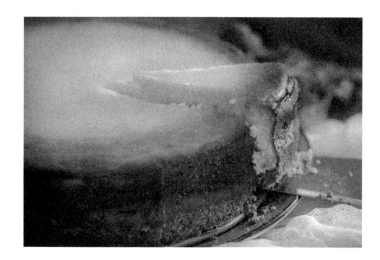

Pistachio Cheesecake

This is a very flavorful cheesecake and is great for the holidays!

1 gluten free graham cracker crust see page 121
16 ounces cream cheese, softened
½ cup sugar
½ cup sour cream
2 teaspoons green food coloring (more if you desire a darker green cheese cake)
½ cup chopped pistachios
2 teaspoons almond extract
2 eggs

Preheat oven to 300°F

Make the crust according to instructions on page 121. Press into the bottom of a spring form pan lined with parchment and both grease parchment and sides of pan or use GF pan spray.
Whip the cream cheese until no lumps remain.
Add the sugar and beat in completely.
Add the sour cream and beat in completely.
Add eggs one at a time and beat well after each egg to make sure it is incorporated completely
Add flavoring and food coloring.
Fold in the nuts.

Pour into a prepared pan and bake at 300 degrees for 1 hour (for 8" Pan, 50 minutes for 10" spring form pan) before opening the door of the oven.

At 1 hour baking time check the cheese cake for doneness and when the outer 2 inches are done and the center appears set, (it may sill jiggle slightly) remove from the oven and run a knife around the outside of the pan.

Place the cake in a warm area to cool. Cool in pan completely.
Cut the cheesecake with a wet, sharp knife for best results and serve with whipped cream.

Polish Christmas Cake

3 cups Kathy's GFFM page 18
1 tablespoon xanthan gum
2 teaspoons baking soda
1 teaspoon allspice
2 cups white sugar (organic or coconut sugar works well too)
1 teaspoon cinnamon
1 teaspoon nutmeg
1 teaspoon cloves
1 teaspoon salt
⅔ cup butter
2 cups buttermilk
1 cup chopped dates and/or raisins
½ cup chopped walnuts

Combine flour, xanthan gum, sugar, baking soda, spices and salt in a bowl. Whisk with a wire whisk to combine.

Cut in butter with a pastry knife or two knives until particles resemble rice kernels

Add buttermilk and mix thoroughly. Mix in dates and nuts

Turn batter onto a generously greased (bottom only) 9 inch tube pan or two 8x4x3 inch loaf pans

Bake at 350 about one hour or until a pick comes out clean when inserted in the center of the cake

Cool in pan on a wire rack for 15 minutes

Remove from pan and cool completely on a wire rack

Flourless Chocolate Cake

This is a Classic French cake. It is also gluten free as there is no flour… very rich and excellent. The quality of the chocolate matters.

Preheat oven to 350 degrees

Prepare 1 9" round cake pan with a parchment circle cut out for the bottom and spray the sides and the parchment circle with GF Pan Spray.

8 ounces of chocolate
½ pound of butter
½ cup of sugar
½ cup of half and half (sometimes I use heavy whipping cream)
1 ½ teaspoon vanilla
¼ teaspoon salt
4 eggs

Heat the butter and cream until bubbles form and then turn off the heat and add the chocolate to melt. Make sure the chocolate is chopped into fine pieces and stir constantly so it is smooth. Let cool while you do the next step.

Whisk eggs, sugar, vanilla and salt,

Temper the chocolate mixture into the egg mixture. This is done by slowly adding the hot liquid into the eggs in a thin steady stream until about half is incorporated. Egg whites cook at 140°F, so if you try to add the hot liquid to the eggs too quickly, you will cook the eggs. This is known as curdling.

Pour into prepared pans and bake at 350 for 25-30 minutes. Insert a toothpick slightly off center, it should come out with fudgy crumbs. The sides should look cooked and dry, similar to a brownie. Do not over bake. Cooking to 165 is sufficient if you want to use a thermometer

Note: when making this gluten free, be careful to check the ingredients for flour. For example, some pan spray releases contain flour.

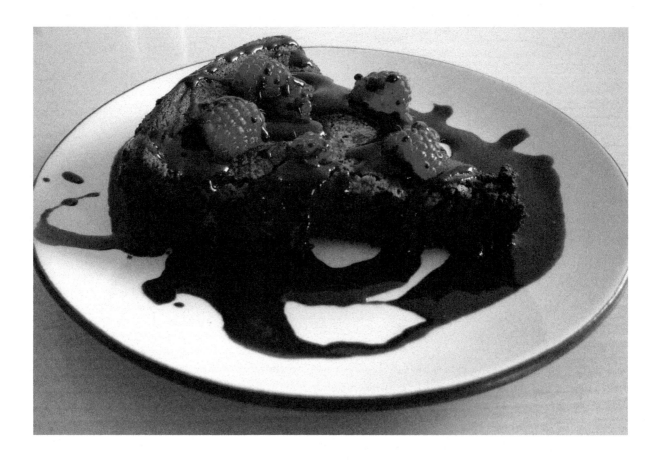

Bread Pudding

I used the White Bread recipe that is in this book to make the bread for the bread pudding. You can use French bread, regular bread, or dinner rolls as long as it is gluten free bread. The White Bread recipe on in this book is a rich dough, so when they were done it was almost like a cinnamon bun it was so rich. Store the finished product in the refrigerator or freezer.

4 eggs
1 cup milk
½ cup sugar
1 tablespoon vanilla
1 teaspoon cinnamon
4 cups gluten free bread, cubed

Preheat oven to 350 degrees. Use a spray release to coat either a 10 inch pie pan or 13x9 inch cake pan,

Mix the first 4 ingredients and add in the bread cubes. Let stand for 15 minutes and then with a wire whisk or potato masher, mash the bread cubes. Mix well and make sure all of the bread is incorporated in. pour into a prepared pie plate or cake pan. It should look really wet with liquid standing around the edges.

Bake at 350 for about 45 minutes until a tester comes out clean or the internal temperature is over 165 degrees, not to exceed 185 though.

Cool slightly and top with hard sauce.

Hard Sauce

2 tablespoons butter
1 tablespoon brandy
¾ cups powdered sugar

Either softened the butter in the microwave or at room temperature. With an electric mixer mix the brandy and butter, add in the powdered sugar until the desired thickness. It should be about the consistency of regular icing. Spread on slightly cooled cake and let it melt in.

Chocolate Texas Sheet Cake

Feel free to serve this cake to everyone! People will not be able to tell it is gluten free. It is that good...

Preheat oven to 350 degrees

Grease and flour 11x17 inch cookie sheet pan

2 sticks margarine*
5 tablespoons cocoa
1 cup water
2 cups Kathy's GFFM page 18
1 teaspoon xanthan gum
1 teaspoon baking soda
2 cups sugar
½ teaspoon salt
½ cup buttermilk or sour milk*
2 slightly beaten eggs
1 teaspoon vanilla

Melt margarine, water and cocoa together and bring to a boil; remove from heat.

Combine flour, baking soda, sugar and salt in mixing bowl and mix with a whisk to combine.

Pour cocoa mixture over the flour mixture and mix until smooth

Add buttermilk, vanilla and eggs, mix well and then beat on medium speed 2 minutes scrape sides and bottom of bowl as needed.

Pour into a prepared cookie sheet and bake for 20- 28 minutes or until pick inserted in center comes out clean.

Frosting

1 stick butter
⅓ cup buttermilk
¼ cup cocoa
2 tablespoons corn syrup
1 pound powdered sugar
½ to 1 cup nuts
1 teaspoon vanilla

Melt margarine, buttermilk, cocoa and syrup and bring to a boil. Remove from heat and add sugar, nuts and vanilla and stir until smooth,

Spread on cake while cake is still warm.

This is an amazing frosting!

*Use almond milk and gluten free dairy free butter substitute for a dairy free cake.

Dark Chocolate Cake

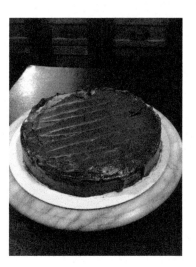

This can be made dairy free also.

Life will not ever be the same! This is an amazing cake. People will not know it is gluten free!

2 cups sugar, white or coconut sugar (if using coconut sugar increase water to 1 ¼ cup and soften the sugar in milk before using)
1 ¾ cups Kathy's GFFM page 18
¾ cup cocoa (I prefer Hershey's)
1 teaspoons xanthan gum
2 teaspoons baking soda
2 teaspoons baking powder
1 teaspoon salt
1 cup milk (Almond Milk if making the cake dairy free)
2 large eggs
¾ cup vegetable oil melted (coconut oil works great too)
2 teaspoons vanilla extract
1 cup boiling water (increase to 1 ¼ cups if using coconut sugar)

Preheat the oven to 350°F.
Prepare 2 9" round baking pans either by greasing with shortening, coconut oil or gluten free pan spray.
Mix all dry ingredients in a stand mixing bowl with a wire whisk.
Put water on to boil.
Mix all wet ingredients except the water.
Add the wet ingredients to the dry ingredients and mix thoroughly.
Beat ingredients on medium speed for 2 minutes.
Stir in boiling water
Pour into prepared pan and bake for 20-25 minutes until tester comes out done.
Cool 10 minutes in pan, turn out and continue to cool on wire rack.

Peanut butter filling

1 cup peanut butter
½ cup brown sugar
4 tablespoons coconut flour (this is specific because of the oils in the peanut butter. The coconut flour is more absorbent and will absorb the excess oil in the peanut butter. You can use regular gluten free flour, but you may need to increase it by a tablespoon or more depending on your taste)

Mix all ingredients and let stand. Spread between 2 layers of chocolate cake or on the top of one cake and top with chocolate sauce.

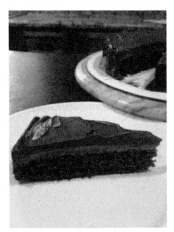

Chocolate frosting

1 stick butter softened
1/3 cup honey
¼ cup cocoa powder
1 teaspoon vanilla

Put all ingredients in a bowl and whip. Spread on cake

This cake is wonderful without the peanut butter filling. Just cover with strawberries and whipping cream and serve. Frosting or no frosting it is a delightful summer treat!

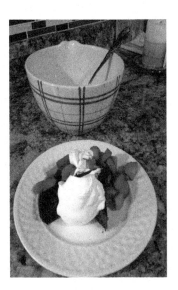

Cherry Pie Filling Cake

This cake is really good and moist. Be careful not to overcook it though.

Pre heat oven to 350 degrees. Lightly grease or spray 9x13 inch pan with a gluten free pan spray

Batter

2 cups Kathy's GFFM page 18
1 teaspoon xanthan gum
1 cup sugar
1 can cherry pie filling (check that it is gluten free)
1 teaspoon baking soda
1 teaspoon baking powder
1 teaspoon vanilla
2 eggs
⅔ cup vegetable oil
¾ cup walnuts (optional)

Mix the flour and xanthan gum and then place all of the remaining ingredients in a large bowl and mix by hand until very well blended. Pour into lightly greased (or spray with spray release) 9X13 inch baking pan

Topping

⅓ cup brown sugar
¼ cup white sugar
1 teaspoon cinnamon
1 cup walnuts

Mix together and sprinkle over the batter before placing in the oven. Bake at 350 degrees for 45 minutes

Chocolate Cherry Cake

This recipe was one of my Aunt Victoria's who was my grandmother's younger sister.

½ cup butter or margarine
1 cup sugar
1 egg
1 square semi-sweet chocolate, melted
1 ½ cup Kathy's GFFM page 18
1 teaspoon xanthan gum
½ teaspoon salt
¼ cup cherry juice
¾ cup buttermilk
1 teaspoon baking soda
15 finely cut cherries (toss the cherries in 2 tablespoons of the flour to prevent them from settling on the bottom of the pan)

Preheat oven to 350 degrees

Grease a 13x9 inch cake pan or spray with a gluten free pan spray.

In the bowl of a stand mixer, cream butter, sugar, egg.

Add the cherry juice then add the melted chocolate, blend well.

Mix the flour, xanthan gum and salt together with a whisk.

Add 1 teaspoon baking soda to the buttermilk and add to the butter mixture alternating with the flour mixture.

Fold the cherries into the cake mixture and bake for 35 minutes or until tester inserted into the center of the cake comes out clean.

Spicy Nuts

3 cups pecan halves
1 cup white sugar
⅓ cup water
1 tablespoons cinnamon
½ teaspoon nutmeg
½ teaspoon salt

Heat sugar, water, cinnamon and nutmeg in sauce pan and boil for 2 minutes stirring continuously. Add the pecans and stir to coat. Then pour onto a cookie sheet lined with parchment. Separate with a fork and let dry. The pecans can be stored in an airtight container at room temperature for up to 2 weeks.

Buttery Nuts

3 cups pecan halves
1 cup white sugar
⅓ cup water
2 teaspoons cinnamon
¼ cup butter

Heat sugar, water, cinnamon and butter in a sauce pan and boil for 2 minutes stirring continuously. Add the pecans and stir to coat. Then pour onto a cookie sheet lined with parchment. Use a fork to separate the nuts and let dry. The pecans can be stored in an airtight container at room temperature for up to 2 weeks.

Fudge

This fudge recipe is a personal favorite. My Grandmother always made it at Christmas. She made peanut butter and chocolate fudge. I now make peanut butter, chocolate, milk chocolate with extra marshmallows… you can make your own special flavor with chocolates, liqueurs… whatever you like. Check all ingredients for gluten free and have fun!

1 12 ounce can evaporated milk (not condensed!)
½ cup (1 stick) butter or margarine
4 cups white sugar
12 ounce bag chocolate chips (or peanut butter chips, milk chocolate chips…)
1 bag of marshmallows (not mini)
1 teaspoon of vanilla or other flavoring
1 cup nuts or additional marshmallows…etc.

Prepare a lined pan 13x9. You can line the pan with parchment paper or grease the pan well with butter or margarine.

In a large pan, cook evaporated milk, butter and sugar to the soft ball stage of 234 degrees. Stir constantly and use a candy thermometer. The milk and milk solids in the butter will scorch easily, stir from the bottom to prevent this.

Remove from the heat and add the chocolate chips, marshmallows and flavoring.

Stir until the marshmallows and chocolate chips are melted.

Add additional chips, nuts, or any other flavoring you desire.

Pour into the prepared pan and allow to set. Cut the fudge before it is completely set.

Store in air tight container in a cool area.

Gluten Free Pie Crust

1 ¼ cup Kathy's GFFM page 18
½ cup millet flour
1 tablespoon sugar (coconut sugar or organic sugar works fine)
1 ½ teaspoons xanthan gum
½ teaspoon salt
6 tablespoons cold butter
1 large egg
2 teaspoons lemon juice

Mix dry ingredient in a mixing bowl with a whisk to make sure they are well blended.

Cut in the cold butter with a pastry knife

Mix the egg and lemon juice together until very foamy and then mix into the dry ingredients. Stir until the mixtures holds together adding additional cold water if necessary.

Shape into a ball and chill for an hour or up to overnight.

Rest the dough for 10 to 15 minutes before working it.

Roll the dough out on a surface that has been heavily dusted with gluten free baking mix or cornstarch. It works best to roll it on plastic wrap so you can pan it easier.

Place the dough into a lightly greased pie pan.

Fill and bake

Graham Cracker Crust

8-9 GF Graham crackers
¼ cup Kathy's GFFM page 18
¼ cup sugar
1 stick margarine

Crush the crackers so that they are really fine. Add the remainder of the ingredients and press into the bottom of the pan you are using.

When using a spring form pan, make sure the crust is over the seam of the bottom and the ring of the pan.

Strawberry Pie

1 pie shell fully cooked or 1 graham cracker crust pressed into a greased pie plate and pre-cooked for 15-20 minutes at 325°F.

Filling

1 quart fresh strawberries, cleaned
1 cup sugar
3 tablespoons corn starch
1 cup water
A few drops of red food coloring

1 pint whipped cream
Chop (or slice as you prefer) all berries.

Place 1 cup of chopped berries in sauce pan with sugar and corn starch.
Add water, a little at a time and cook and stir until thick and clear. Add food coloring and stir the mixture and let it cool.

After the mixture cools, add the remaining cut berries and place in baked pie shell.
Top with whipped cream and refrigerate.
Refrigerate

Apple Pie Filling

1 pie crust from page 120
¼ cup Kathy's GFFM page 18
⅓ cup white sugar (coconut sugar or organic sugar works fine);
½ teaspoon ground nutmeg;
½ teaspoon ground cinnamon.
Dash of salt
8 cups thinly sliced pared tart apples

Peel apples, core and slice thin and place them in lemon juice and water. This will prevent browning.

Mix flour, sugar, nutmeg, cinnamon and salt and toss in the apples.

Topping

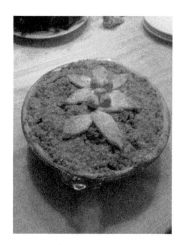

1 teaspoon cinnamon
1 cup gluten free rolled oats (quick cooking, not steel cut)
¾ cup Gluten free multipurpose flour
¾ cup brown sugar
½ cup butter

Mix the cinnamon, oats, flour and sugar. Cut in the butter.
Press this topping onto the apples, patting it in.

Bake at 350 for about 50 to 60 minutes.

Lemon Crunch Pie

This pie is best made the day before and kept covered in the refrigerator overnight or you can serve it the day you make it. When serving the day you make it, just give it a couple hours to set in the refrigerator before serving. Use Key Lime juice instead of Lemon juice for another variety of this pie.

1 pie shell fully cooked from page 120.

Filling

1 can sweetened condensed milk (not evaporated)
¾ cup lemon juice (½ cup if you do not like a tart pie)
5 egg yolks
1 teaspoon vanilla
2 tablespoons butter
2 tablespoons sugar
½ cup Kathy's GFFM page 18

Preheat oven to 325°F.

Mix the sugar and Kathy's GFFM in a bowl and cut in the butter until small clumps form (about the size of raw peas). Set aside.

With a wire whisk, mix the sweetened condensed milk and egg yolks until completely mixed in. Add the lemon juice and vanilla and continue to mix with the whisk until completely mixed in.

Pour into the cooked pie shell and crumble the flour and butter mixture over the pie filling.

Bake for 20 minutes.

Remove from oven and let cool.

Apple Strudel

This is fantastic. This pastry can also be used as a pie crust, crust for meat pies… it is very versatile.

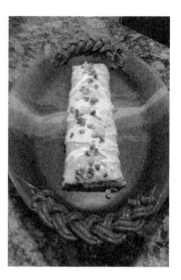

Pastry:
1 ¼ cups Kathy's GFFM page 18
¼ cup millet flour
¼ cup sweet sorghum flour
4 teaspoons xanthan gum
1 teaspoon unflavored gelatin
1 egg
¼ cup milk (you can use almond milk if dairy free)
1 stick butter, melted. (use gluten free/dairy free butter substitute to make it dairy free)
1 tablespoon raw honey.

Add the gelatin to the cold milk to dissolve. Warm the milk slightly after the gelatin has dissolved.

Melt the butter. Do this step in the beginning so that it has a chance to begin cooling.

In a large bowl, mix the flours and xanthan gum.

Mix the milk, warm butter (not hot), honey and egg and add to the dry ingredients. Mix with a fork or wooden spoon until well incorporated. The dough should be soft, but not sticky. Should it be too dry, add a little more milk.

With your hands, gather the dough and squeeze into a ball. Wrap in plastic wrap until you are ready to use it. You can refrigerate it should you not need it right away, just be sure to let it warm to room temperature before rolling it out.

Apple Filling:

4 apples, peeled, cored and chopped in large chunks
½ cup apple juice
½ cup water
1 teaspoon unflavored gelatin
1 teaspoon lemon juice
2 tablespoons sugar (for cooking apples)
¼ teaspoon cinnamon (for cooking apples)
¼ teaspoon nutmeg (for cooking apples)
1 tablespoon sugar
1 teaspoon cinnamon

Add the gelatin to the water and let stand to soften the gelatin while you peel the apples.

In a medium sauce pan, combine apples, apple juice with gelatin, water, sugar and spices and lemon juice. Bring to a boil and then cook for about 8-10 minutes until the apples are tender.

Separate the dough into half. Wrap the half not using and refrigerate for later use or freeze it for longer storage.

Roll the dough out on a full sheet of parchment roll out thinly, about 1/8 inch thick. Roll in the shape of a rectangle. Get the width first, then length.

Sprinkle with the cinnamon sugar.

Spoon the cooked apples onto the center of the dough. Use a slotted spoon so that you do not get the liquid that it was cooked in. Using the parchment to fold the pastry, fold 1/3 over the apples.

Fold the other side over then using the parchment, roll the pastry seam side down to bake.

Using a knife, score the top of the pastry to allow the steam to escape. Bake at 350°F for 25-30 minutes until browned. Sprinkle with cinnamon sugar or a glaze made with ½ cup powdered sugar, 1 tablespoon maple syrup and ¼ teaspoon vanilla.

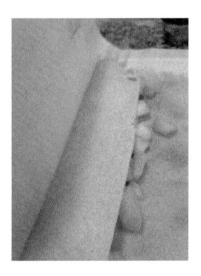

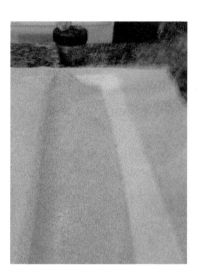

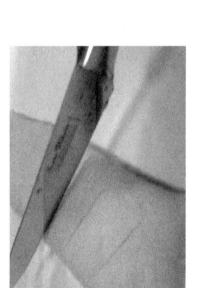

Strawberry Romanoff

This is fantastic! For Holiday parties or special events. Try serving in a martini glass or in a Margaretta glass to upscale this dessert

1 pound sour cream (this is a normal size tub as sold in the grocery store)
¼ cup dark brown sugar
¼ cup light brown sugar
1 tablespoon cinnamon
1 ½ teaspoon nutmeg
½ cup brandy
Whole fresh strawberries

Mix sour cream, sugars, spices and brandy and refrigerate.

Carefully wash strawberries and serve them whole with the sauce in a small dish for dipping or slice and place in the bottom of serving dish (or glass). Top with sauce.

Maple Pound Cake

This is a very rich and moist cake.

1 cup Kathy's GFFM page 18
½ cup millet flour
¼ cup sorghum Flour
¼ cup tapioca flour
1 tablespoon xanthan gum
1 teaspoon baking powder
½ teaspoon baking soda
1 teaspoon salt
¾ cup butter, softened (or butter substitute)
⅔ cup brown sugar, packed
2 large eggs
½ cup amber maple syrup
1 cup sour cream
2 teaspoons vanilla extract

Preheat the oven to 350°F. Grease the bottom and sides of a Bundt pan, or use a gluten free pan spray.

In a medium bowl, combine the flours, baking powder, baking soda and salt. Whisk the ingredients to blend completely.

In the bowl of a stand mixer, beat the butter and sugar until light and fluffy. Add the eggs one at a time and beat until completely mixed in. Stop the mixer and scrape the sides of the bowl as necessary. Add the maple syrup and mix well.

Add the flour mixture and then the sour cream and vanilla. Mix until completely combined, stopping the mixer and scraping the sides and bottom of the pan as necessary.

Spoon mixture into the Bundt pan and smooth the top.

Let stand 10 minutes.

Bake 50-60 minutes until tester inserted into the center of the cake comes out clean.

Cool for 10 minutes before removing from the pan.

While cake is cooling make the glaze

Maple Glaze Frosting

1 cup powdered sugar
⅛ cup (2 tablespoons) amber maple syrup
2 Tablespoons water

Mix all ingredients with a whisk in a bowl and drizzle over the cake while still hot.

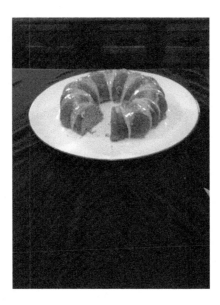

Shortcakes

2 ⅓ cups Kathy's GFFM page 18
1 ½ teaspoons xanthan gum
¼ cup sugar
⅓ cup butter (or gluten free butter substitute if you are dairy free)
¾ cups milk (use almond milk if you are dairy free)
3 eggs beaten
1 teaspoon vanilla
4 cups strawberries
1 tablespoon sugar
1 cup whipping cream
1 tablespoon sugar
1 teaspoon vanilla

Carefully wash the strawberries and chop them into the size you prefer. Place them in a large bowl and top with 1 tablespoon sugar. Stir and refrigerate so they release their juices.

Heat oven to 450°F. Grease a cookie sheet.

In medium bowl combine flour mix, xanthan gum and sugar, stir with a whisk.

Cut in the butter with a pastry knife. Stir in milk, eggs and vanilla.

Portion out onto cookie sheet, generally makes 6 but you can make them smaller if you wish.

Bake 10-12 minutes or until light golden brown.

Whip the cream until soft peaks form. Add the sugar and vanilla and continue whipping until stiff peaks form.

Let the shortcakes cool at least 5 minutes and then split and top with strawberries and whipped cream.

Éclair and Cream Puff Dough (Pate Choux Paste and Pastry Cream Recipes)

The next 3 pages are dedicated to a classic that is just as good gluten free!

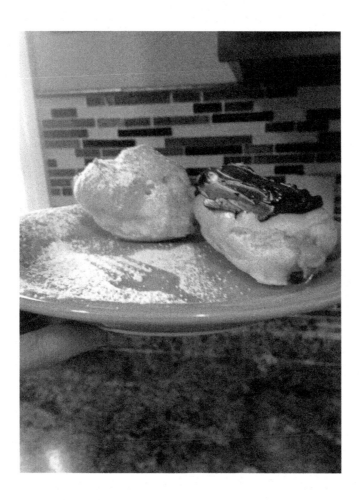

Gluten Free Pate Choux Paste (Éclair and cream puff shells)

1 cup water
½ cup butter or dairy free butter substitute
¼ teaspoon salt
1 cup Kathy's GFFM page 18
½ teaspoon xanthan gum
4 eggs

Heat the oven to 450°F. Line a baking sheet with parchment paper and set aside.

Combine flour and xanthan gum (unless using another flour blend that has xanthan gum in it) in a bowl and whisk to combine

In heavy sauce pan combine water, butter and salt and bring to a rolling boil.

Reduce heat

Add the flour all at once and stir constantly with a wooden spoon until it forms cohesive dough. Cook for 1 to 2 minutes. A film will develop on the bottom of the pan and some of the oil will separate out and that is fine.

Transfer to a stand mixer and beat at medium speed until the dough temperate reaches between 120 and 130 degrees.

Add eggs one at a time, incorporating each egg completely before adding the next egg. Once all eggs are incorporated, mix the dough on medium speed for 5 minutes.

Let dough rest for 5 minutes.

Either pipe éclairs with a pastry bag with a large round piping tip or a disposable bag with the end cut to allow you to pipe about 1 inch round and 5 inch long éclairs. You can either pipe the cream puffs or use a portion scoop to make the rounds. Remember they will puff in size so a 2 ounce scoop is large when cooked. You can make them smaller or larger as you prefer, just adjust cooking times appropriately.

Cook in oven for approximately 20 minutes at 450°F then reduce the oven and cook for 15-20 additional minutes at 375F until done. They should be browned and sound hollow when tapped. Not cooking them long enough will cause them to collapse when cooling. Using a skewer or chop stick, puncture a hole on each side of the éclair to allow steam to escape. Should a hole naturally form during the cooking process, it is not necessary to puncture the ends. Puncture the sides of the cream puffs too.

Turn off oven and leave in the oven with the door open for 5 additional minutes.

Cool completely before filling. These can be frozen for use later. You can place back in a 450°F oven for a few minutes to re-crisp if desired.

Gluten Free Pastry Cream

The eclairs pictured are made with coconut sugar and that is why the filling is light brown in color. You can use white sugar if you prefer. Using white sugar will produce the bright yellow pastry cream you are used to seeing.

2 cups milk *(you can use coconut milk if dairy free)*
½ cup white sugar *(you can use coconut sugar if you prefer)*
¼ teaspoon salt
6 egg yolks
3 tablespoons corn starch
2 teaspoons vanilla

Combine milk, sugar and salt in a heavy sauce pan and bring to a boil.

Whisk egg yolks until frothy.

Sift the cornstarch over the eggs and mix in.

Temper the milk mixture into the egg mixture. Tempering is adding the hot milk in a thin stream using a ladle so that you do not curdle the eggs. Yolks cook at 165 degrees and any egg whites that are in there from separating cook at 148-158 degrees. Cooling the milk mixture slightly while you whisk the eggs and add the cornstarch will help along with the tempering. You want to raise the temperate of the eggs slowly to prevent them cooking (or called curdling)

After adding about ½ to ¾ of the milk to the eggs, add the egg mixture to the remainder of the milk in the pan and return to the stove. With the heat on medium, cook, stirring continuously, until the mixture gets thick and begins to boil. Turn the heat down and continue to cook for 1-2 minutes to cook the corn starch. Do not allow it to come to a rolling boil, just a soft boil. Do not cook longer than 2 minutes. Set a timer.

Turn off and add vanilla. Stir to incorporate the vanilla

Pour into a 13x9" cake pan to cool. Cover with plastic wrap, putting the wrap directly on the pastry cream to prevent skin from forming.

Cool slightly and refrigerate. Do not leave at room temperature! Once this reaches 145 degrees it needs to be held in the refrigerator.

Once the éclairs have cooled either pipe the filling into the éclairs or remove the top and fill with the filling and replace the top.

Top with powdered sugar or chocolate glaze.

Chocolate Glaze

⅔ cup chocolate chips (gluten free and if necessary, dairy free)
½ cup heavy cream (you can use coconut creamer for dairy free)
½ teaspoon vanilla (make sure that your vanilla is gluten free, not all vanilla is)

Bring cream (or coconut creamer) to slight boil and pour over chocolate chips. Let stand 5 minutes to melt chocolate. Stir and add the vanilla. Stir and let cool. Spread on the éclairs and store the remaining topping in the refrigerator.

Index

CPSIA information can be obtained
at www.ICGtesting.com
Printed in the USA
FSOW04n1522030117
29157FS